PERSONAL TRAINER
BODY MASSAGE

ESME FLOYD
WITH PAUL WILLS

CARLTON
BOOKS

THIS IS A CARLTON BOOK

Text, design and special photography
copyright © 2004 Carlton Books Limited

First published in 2004
This edition published in 2010
by Carlton Books Limited
20 Mortimer Street
London W1T 3JW

ISBN 978 1 84732 474 0

Printed and bound in Dubai

Senior Executive Editor: **Lisa Dyer**
Copy Editors: **Lol Henderson and Lara Maiklem**
Art Editor: **Vicky Holmes**
Designer: **Penny Stock**
Production Controller: **Lisa Moore**
Photographer: **Anna Stevenson**
Models: **Suzanne Burnett, Nicole Le Grange
and Sage Peakson**
Indexer: **Diana LeCore**

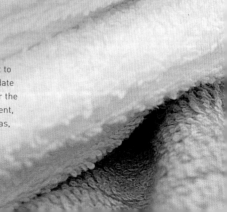

CONTENTS

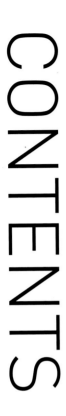

Introduction

The healing touch of massage is one of the best gifts you can give your body. It has been used in human societies for thousands of years as one of the principle therapies for both mind and body healing. Massage is not only an aid for relaxing away stress and tension and stimulating healing, it also boosts circulation and helps tired bodies to rejuvenate themselves, ready for the rigours of everyday life.

All too often we take our bodies for granted, asking them to work all day with little or no reward. Learning to use massage can give your body the special treat it needs and help you to thank it for everything it gives you. This book will show you how to give your friends and family all the benefits of a professional massage in the privacy of your own home and how to use your own healing touch to solve body problems and ease stress, once and for all.

This book is designed to show you how to share the caring and healing touch of massage with your partner, friends and family. It should also help you to develop your own unique massage style by encouraging you to create your own sequences. It is a complete guide, covering techniques for the back, neck and shoulders, the arms and legs and the abdomen. It is intended to show you how to give a total body massage that will help you to relax and unwind. Self-massage techniques are also explained, showing how to combat common illnesses and injuries, to soothe away pain and de-stress in minutes.

Massage has benefits, not only for the receiver but also for the giver. It encourages closeness and caring, boosts body awareness by the power of touch and teaches the hands to 'hear' the body beneath them. It gives you emotional 'time out', allowing you to focus entirely on the massage and how it makes you feel, boosting self-awareness and revitalizing the mind-body connection. The soothing strokes and deep breathing techniques discourage worry and stress and give the giver and receiver the chance to get in touch with their real feelings.

To help you to use massage in the right way, each of the techniques in this book is designed to stand alone. The individual techniques are also arranged in sequence so that they can be used to perform a whole body massage. From this, you can choose how to make the best use of the book: dip in and out to target specific areas; concentrate on a few techniques for a quick fix if you're short of time; or go slowly and follow the techniques through from beginning to end for a total all-over body massage.

All the techniques here are explained for one side of the body only; to perform the technique on the other side, simply reverse the instructions and repeat. It is usual for massage therapists to concentrate on one side of the body at a time, working through all the massages on one side before working on the other. The method prevents too much movement around the body and allows the masseur to maintain smoothness and fluidity throughout the massage.

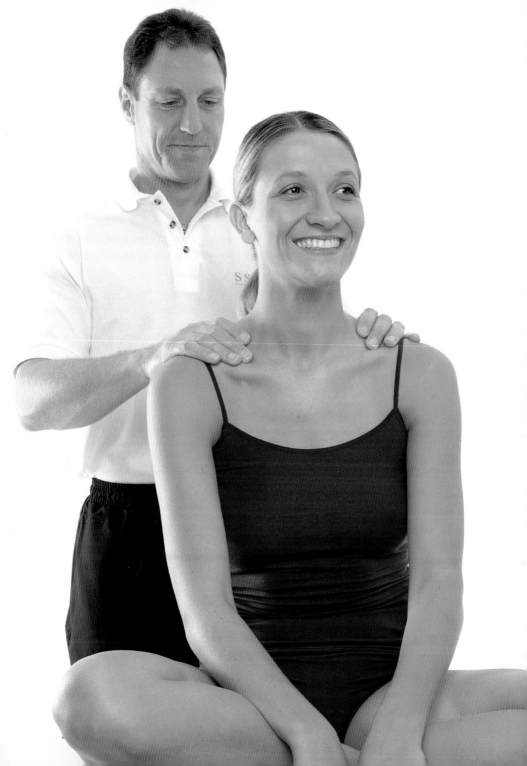

Understanding
Massage

Massage has been used for centuries to heal, invigorate and relax the mind and body, reaching all the major organs as well as helping the muscles, bones and soft tissue stay healthy.

The massage principle is simple: touch means stimulation. This means that wherever touch is used, the body reacts. Because of the changing landscape of the skin and the body parts it protects, differing levels of touch on the body elicit a range of responses; a soft stroke of the forearm may induce relaxation, but a deeper touch might help the blood vessels in the lower arm take blood back to the heart or stimulate and deepen blood flow to painful muscles.

It is important that anyone using massage, even if it is just at home, has a basic understanding of how it works on different areas of the body. This chapter will help you understand some of the fundamental principles, techniques and benefits of massage.

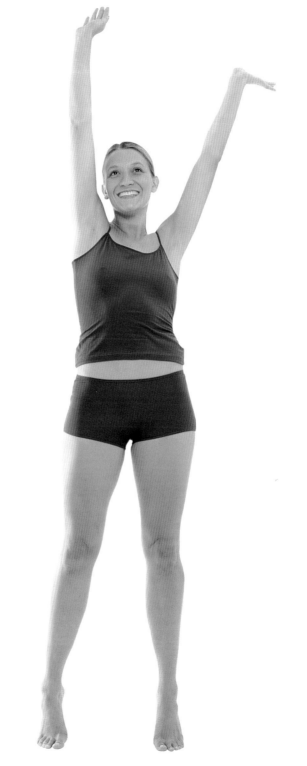

Helping your body

In order for our bodies to work efficiently, the many complex systems that exist under our skin have to work together in a coordinated way. Bones, muscles and soft tissues help us to move. A circulatory system consisting of heart, lungs arteries and blood allows oxygen to be transported around the body to keep cells alive. The nervous system keeps the brain informed of what's going on and allows us to think, act and feel. Our digestive system helps us absorb energy from food and keeps us hydrated with water. An immune system prevents attack from viruses, bacteria and other micro-organisms that could cause us harm or spread disease.

Massage can help each of these systems work optimally, boosting general health and wellbeing and encouraging healing and growth, right down to a microscopic level.

Bones, muscles and soft tissues

Thanks to our skeletal system, the network of bones and of soft tissues that surround them, our bodies are capable of an amazing range of movements. The effects of massage on the skeletal system are long term – they continue to work long after the actual massage ends, stimulating healing and repair of soft tissue adhesions for up to a month afterwards.

Muscles are made up of bundles of fibres that glide over each other and contract to generate movement. Muscles are attached to bones by tendons and bones are attached to each other by ligaments. Muscle fibres only work in one direction – that is, they contract to shorten themselves but cannot extend. This is why, all around the body, muscles are arranged in opposing pairs so that as one contracts the other expands to

allow movement in all directions. Muscles, tendons and ligaments can all be affected by adhesions and small scars or tears that create sore spots. These can stop the tissues from working properly, and can also become severe if left untreated. Massage helps to break down these adhesions.

Circulation

Massage not only stimulates the general circulation system of the body, but it also boosts circulation at a very localized level. Our bodies are made up of thousands of cells and every one of them needs a regular supply of blood. Blood brings all the ingredients the cells need for growth, nutrition and repair; it also takes away waste products and toxins. Massage stimulates the flow of blood and boosts the supply of nutrients – such as minerals and vitamins for health and sugar for energy – and the removal of toxins.

Lymphatic drainage

The body has another, separate, circulatory system that transports a fluid called lymph around the body via a series of glands and vessels. Impurities and toxins are filtered through the glands (called lymph nodes) and the clean fluid drains back into the bloodstream. This helps the immune system by removing bacteria, viruses and other foreign matter, thus fighting infection and draining away excess fluid. Damaged or stiff tissues can become thick and fibrous, causing blockage of the pores and affecting lymph drainage. Massage helps fluids to travel towards the heart and also stimulates muscle contractions that remove fluid blockages. Lymphatic drainage is one of the reasons that all the techniques in this book – and all good massage therapists – work from the outside of the body in towards the heart.

Nervous system

There are two nervous systems that run throughout the body. The first, the sympathetic nervous system, responds to pressure, touch, temperature and so on, passing messages to the brain and responding to sensory stimulation. The second, the parasympathetic nervous system, is the unconscious system that controls body functions, such as heart rate, liver function, digestion and metabolism – the 'behind the scenes' mechanisms that work constantly to keep you alive. Massage stimulates both of the nervous systems, working on the sympathetic system's nerve endings and receptors in the skin and muscles to reduce tension and overactivity and also the parasympathetic nervous system, having a positive effect on conditions such as abnormal blood pressure, digestive disorders, migraine and insomnia.

Skin

The skin is the body's largest organ, providing a flexible protective covering to all body parts, giving us shape and holding us together, containing body fluids and acting as the first line of defence against injury and invasion by bacteria, viruses and microbes. There are three main layers – the upper, epidermis; the middle, dermis; and the lower, subcutaneous.

The epidermis, which is the visible, outer layer of skin, is constantly regenerating itself, producing new cells in the lower layers that rise to the surface and are eventually shed. The dermis lies directly underneath the epidermis and is filled with a rich supply of blood vessels, lymph, nerve endings, sweat and oil glands and hair follicles. The subcutaneous layer lies beneath the dermis and provides a storage facility for fat, which acts as a heat insulator and also provides a protective layer. Massage boosts circulation in all three layers of skin, encouraging renewal, growth and repair, preventing build-up of dead skin cells and stimulating sweat glands to remove waste products and clear out the pores. It gives the skin a healthy glow and promotes cellular healing at every level.

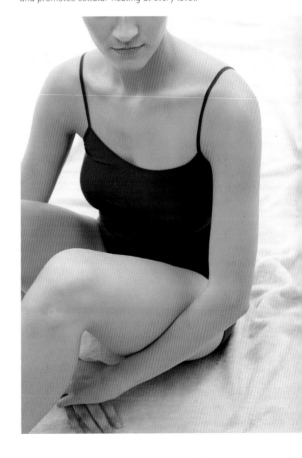

RIGHT **By stimulating circulation, massage boosts the health of the skin.**

Cautions and contraindications

Qualified massage therapists use a range of techniques to treat different problems. The purpose of this book is to give you a general understanding of the therapeutic effects of massage and how you can use it to help yourself, your family and friends to relax and unwind. If you have health problems, always consult a professional before massage.

Massage is generally considered to be an extremely safe form of therapy, but even so there are a few situations in which it might do more harm than good. Several conditions – known as contraindications – are adversely affected by massage. Check before you start that your massage partner is not suffering from any of these and if you have any doubts about safety DO NOT MASSAGE. If you're worried, you'll be tense and won't give a good massage – it's better to wait and seek professional advice, and then you may be able to go ahead with no worries at a later date.

Never give a massage if the person to be massaged has any of the following:

Inflammation

Never massage over inflamed or sore soft tissues because it could make them worse. Look for bruising, swelling, tender or sore muscles or areas of skin, heat and redness in the skin, or pain and dysfunction in the affected area. Swollen or sore lymph nodes (in the neck, underarms and groin) are to be avoided. If you are in doubt, try the ten-second test – apply enough pressure to the area to cause mild discomfort and maintain it for ten seconds. If discomfort decreases it's probably safe to treat, but if it increases you should wait until the inflammation has died down.

Bone and joint injuries

Avoid conditions affecting the bones and joints after injury (like whiplash, fractures, sprains and strains) because massage could aggravate the condition and cause pain.

Open wounds

You should never massage over an open wound because of the risk of infection.

Fever

People develop a high temperature when their bodies are working hard to deal with some sort of infection. Massage is not recommended for people with a temperature over 37.5°C (99.4°F) because it could jeopardize the body's defence systems by raising their temperature further.

Thrombosis

People with a history of thrombosis should not be massaged because it could encourage a clot to come loose and enter the blood. Great care should be taken with conditions known to increase thrombosis risk such as recent major surgery, varicose veins, heart disease, impact trauma, some contraceptive pills and long periods of immobility or bed rest, which reduces circulation. If you are at all concerned or worried, seek medical advice before starting a massage.

Varicose veins

A breakdown in the one-way valves of the veins in the legs causes blood to collect in the veins and gives them a blue, slightly lumpy appearance, known as varicose veins. In many cases, a light stroking over the vein will not do any harm, but deep techniques should be avoided in the leg area as they could exert pressure on already weakened vein walls, causing further problems.

Skin disorders

Disorders like psoriasis, eczema and acne can be aggravated by massage, which should also be avoided in cases of bacterial, fungal or viral infections. You should also avoid other skin problems like cold sores, blisters, sunburn, cuts and grazes, bites, stings and unexplained lumps.

Cancer

Although a trained therapist can sometimes lessen pain and tension caused by cancer, there is a risk that tumours may be spread through the body or that it might be painful. Stick to gentle stroking or consult a doctor.

Drugs and alcohol

Never give a massage to anyone who is under the influence of drugs or alcohol. These are mind- and body-altering substances that can cause people to react in an unpredictable way.

Long-term medical conditions

Although not necessarily contraindications, you should seek medical advice before massaging someone with a long-term condition like epilepsy, severe asthma, oedema, heart disease, chronic back pain, and those on long-term medication.

Other concerns

In addition, there are several other conditions that can have a bearing on the massage you choose to give. Look out for:

Diabetes

The condition can affect circulation in the feet and lower legs, and create fragile tissues that may be damaged by deep massage techniques. Sometimes massage appears to have the same effect on blood sugar levels as exercise, so diet and medication might need altering.

High or low blood pressure

Massage can cause fluctuations in blood pressure levels so be careful around people with high or low blood pressure. If you are at all concerned, seek medical advice first.

Osteoporosis

This disease is a brittle bone condition in which the bones (particularly in the back, neck and shoulders) become thin and easily broken. Deep massage techniques could cause fractures in people with severe osteoporosis, so seek medical advice.

Pregnancy

The aches and pains of pregnancy can be soothed away with the correct massage techniques, reducing swelling and pain and boosting wellbeing. However, massage should be avoided during the first 12 weeks – particularly around the stomach – when the risk of miscarriage and foetal disorders are greatest. Occasionally pregnant women go on to develop conditions like diabetes and high blood pressure, which could contraindicate massage (see above), or they might suffer severe nausea as a result of massage so they should be made aware of this before a session. Essential oils should not be used during pregnancy.

Children and the elderly

Both children and the elderly can benefit greatly from massage, but should not be massaged using deep techniques because they have less lean tissue and could therefore suffer pain or discomfort, and may be less likely to tell you how they feel. Being aware of how much pressure you are exerting and making sure you have a continued dialogue can help to make the massage a beneficial experience for both of you.

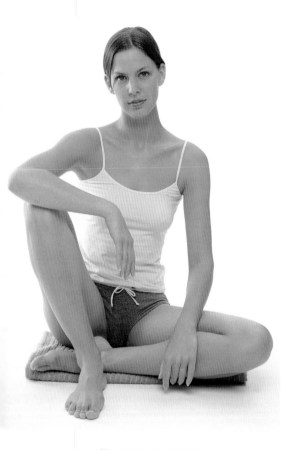

Areas to avoid

There are several places on the body where massage should not be performed under any circumstances. These are:

Eyes – The eyes are delicate and can be damaged by pressure, so avoid pressing or massaging in or around the eyes.

Sides of the neck – The side of the neck holds the carotid artery, which takes oxygen and nutrients to the brain. Pressure here can interrupt blood flow, causing faintness or dizziness and even unconsciousness. Avoid pressing hard on the sides of the neck and be careful around the backs of the ears.

Back of the knees – Behind the knee and slightly above it, there is a soft triangle of tissue that sits between the muscles of the hamstrings as they meet the knee where arteries and veins travel very close to the surface. Leg massages always concentrate on working around this area and never actually on it.

Babies' heads – The plates of a baby's skull are not fully formed for the first two or three years of life and extreme care should be taken when touching these soft areas, called the fontanelles, as well as any part of the neck and face.

Stomach in pregnancy – The stomach and abdomen of pregnant women should be avoided and extreme caution taken with massage in the lower back.

Checklist of contraindications to massage:
- Swelling or Inflammation
- Fever
- Open Wounds
- Bone and Joint Injuries
- Bleeding Disorders
- Melanoma (skin cancer)
- High Blood Pressure
- Cancer
- Varicose Veins
- Deep Vein Thrombosis
- Skin Infections

The benefits of massage for body and mind

One of the most profound benefits of massage is deep relaxation, reducing the stress and tension that is believed to be, directly or indirectly, the cause of nearly three-quarters of all illness. Every single nerve in our bodies, including thousands in the skin, send messages to the brain, which is the control room of the nervous system. It monitors everything that goes on in our bodies as well as our moods and feelings. In this way, touch is linked to emotions, and that's why massage can help beat stress.

Coping with stress

When you are faced with a stressful situation – whether it's an immediate problem like an emergency or a long-term build-up of stress like trouble at work or tiredness – your body responds by secreting the stress hormones adrenaline and cortisol into the bloodstream. These hormones give us the famous 'fight or flight' response that is designed to allow our bodies to react to dangerous situations. When they are released, our muscles tense, ready to spring into action, and the heart and lungs work harder to pump oxygen to the arms and legs. Blood pressure, breathing and pulse rate rise, and oxygenated blood is diverted away from the stomach (halting digestion and causing the 'nervous' sensation of butterflies), the skin (causing it to turn pale), the immune system and organs like the liver and kidneys.

Our bodies are designed to respond to stress – it is only when stressful situations become prolonged that the body starts to suffer damage. Being in a constant state of alertness raises blood pressure and heart rate, and can cause problems with skin, digestion, migraine, back pain and heart disease. Massage helps to combat the harmful effects of long-term stress because it allows the body to slow down and reduces the effects of the stress hormones. It slows breathing and relaxes muscles, which prevent more adrenaline and cortisol from being released into the bloodstream, and simultaneously stimulate the skin and major organs to boost circulation and lymphatic drainage around the whole body.

Time out and general wellbeing

One of the primary benefits of massage is that it gives you time to unwind and be with your thoughts, away from the strains of everyday life. Peaceful surroundings and a calming atmosphere allow the mind time out to relax and recharge. The soothing touch of massage, alongside the space to concentrate, helps to reconnect the mind-body links that can be lost through busy lifestyles. This enables your physical and emotional sides to work together to combat future stress.

The feeling of physical contact stimulates the release of endorphins – also known as feel-good chemicals – in the brain. These lift the mood, help fight pain, boost self-esteem and dissolve the effects of stress, which allow the immune system and major organs to return to functioning normally. Massage reminds your body of the pleasure of taking time out and helps to reduce blood pressure, breathing rate and stress.

The nervous system controls tension in the entire body, which is why nonphysical pressures, such as stress, can lead to physical symptoms like digestive problems and headaches. Massage helps by affecting the nerves to reduce tension and thus increase positive input to the body's systems.

Getting Ready
for Massage

2

Massage is a totally natural therapy that you can do anywhere, at any time and without any specialized equipment. However, because massage is about the mind as well as the body, and because we are affected by everything around us all the time, it is important to create the best possible environment before you start.

This chapter will take you through a few important technical points, such as which massage mediums to use, how to choose aromatherapy oils for their essential oil properties and the best way to use towels to warm, cover and comfort the person you are massaging. It also explains how to create an atmosphere for your massage that gives you a total sensory experience.

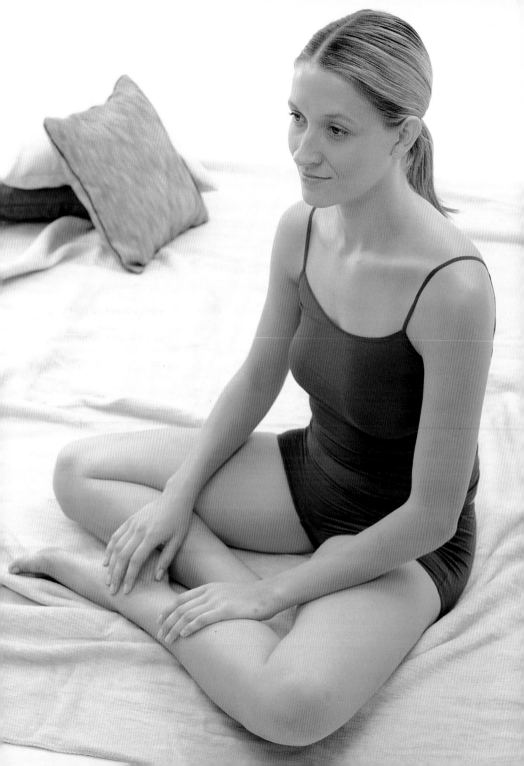

Massage mediums

In order to massage correctly, you need to make sure that your hands can glide over the skin, exerting just the right amount of pressure. To do this, you will need to use a massage medium to reduce frictional drag and to lubricate the surface of the skin. The massage medium you use depends on the skin type of the person being massaged. Skins differ greatly in the amount of oils, lotions and other mediums they absorb, so it's wise to have a few different types ready to use. It is about personal choice, so try a few before you decide which one works best for you and the person you are massaging – trust yourself and choose the one that feels right.

Lotions

Body massage lotions are a combination of oil and cream, which is good for massage because it doesn't absorb too quickly into the skin and can therefore be used sparsely. Lotions are also kind to the therapist's hands, keeping them well moisturized. Massage lotions differ from normal body lotions, which do not contain oil, so they last longer on the skin and are therefore better for massage. Some body massage lotions contain lanolin, which some people are allergic to, so most massage therapists opt for hypoallergenic lotions. Lotions are often the first choice for therapeutic massage, which requires a combination of light and deep strokes.

Creams

Excellent for massaging small areas with light contact, creams moisturize but have high levels of base oil, which means they can become slippery on larger areas. Hand and foot cream and moisturizers containing urea, which doesn't absorb as quickly as other constituents, are particularly good.

Talcum powder

Talc allows a large range of contact with minimal movement and retains a high degree of the natural friction between skin surfaces. It allows for some movement, but also means that the masseur can achieve deeper contact for correctional and friction work. It is a great alternative for people who are allergic to oils, creams and lotions and is more likely to be chosen by a professional for deep work on specific areas than for general massage.

Oils

These do not absorb into the skin very well, which means they are good for light contact, especially if you are working with children, the elderly or people with whom you want to avoid deep contact. The less oil you use, the deeper the contact; the lighter contact you require, the more oil you need, but remember the skin surface should never be so slippery that you are not in control of your strokes. Oils differ in absorption but most commonly available massage oils will be light oils, which are good for a soft, relaxing massage.

Aromatherapy oils

Essential oils can be combined with a base carrier oil, such as almond, to further the therapeutic benefits of the massage.

Caution: Essential oils are potent and can be harmful if misused, so always follow the manufacturer's instructions. Obtain oils from a reputable source and dilute in the right proportions. With the exception of lavender and tea tree, no undiluted essential oils should be applied directly onto the skin, and oils should never be eaten, drunk or applied to lips and eyes. Essential oils should be avoided in pregnancy – especially in the first 12 weeks – and help should be sought from a qualified practitioner before using them on children and the elderly. Many stores now sell ready-mixed massage oils, but the following essential oils are commonly used:

Lavender – Sleep-inducing, calming and antidepressant. May help: headaches, skin complaints, stretchmarks, high and low blood pressure, muscular pains, rheumatism and arthritis. An excellent carrier oil because of its beneficial effects.

Black pepper – Warming, stimulating and invigorating. May help: stiff and tired muscles and joints, sluggish circulation, decreased mobility. May irritate some skins.

Camomile – Sedative, antidepressant and sleep-inducing. May help: high blood pressure, general aches and pains, dry skin and eczema. Approved as safe for use with children because of its mildness, it is also good for using on the elderly.

Marjoram – Sedative, circulation-boosting and warming. May help: sore and tired muscles, joint pains, headaches and arthritis. Marjoram should not be used in combination with clary sage, as the mixture could be potentially intoxicating.

BELOW **Oils, creams and lotions have different textures and absorbabilities.**

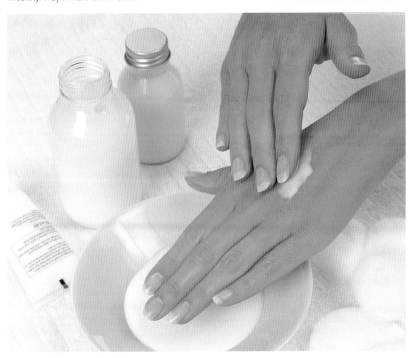

Orange and Grapefruit – Uplifting, stimulating and antidepressant. May help: depression, sluggishness and lack of motivation.

Bergamot – Antidepressant, mood-boosting and balancing. May help: depression, anxiety and winter blues. Bergamot is phototoxic, so exposure to the sun and sunbeds should be avoided for 12 hours afterwards.

Rose – Calming, antidepressant and a general body tonic. May help: insomnia and dry skin conditions.

Frankincense – Mentally stimulating and boosts self-awareness. May help: meditation, concentration and self-reflection.

Sandalwood – Confidence-boosting, anti-inflammatory, sedative and boosts the immune system. May help: low self-esteem, sciatic pain and dry skin.

Tea tree – Antiviral, antiseptic, fungicidal and boosts the immune system. May help: promote healing, reduce swelling and fight off infection.

Eucalyptus – Immune-boosting and a decongestant. May help: sinus problems, coughs and colds, and chest infections. Eucalyptus can produce erythema in some people.

Rosemary – Memory boosting and mentally stimulating. May help: stimulate memory and brain activity, prepare your brain for exams, presentations, speeches, etc.

For stress: Try combining lavender, bergamot and camomile.

For aching muscles: Try using lavender, black pepper and marjoram.

For an energy boost: Try lavender, rosemary and grapefruit or orange.

For depression: Try lavender, eucalyptus and peppermint.

If you're using essential oils for massage, don't have an oil burner, scented candle or perfume in the room as they could interact. Also, don't combine more than three scents in one carrier oil. You should never use an oil if either of you dislike the smell.

Towelling

Several purposes are served by towelling. First, it provides barriers – the person being massaged knows the physical limitations of your massage and that it will not go beyond the barrier of the towel – this is essential to ensure that they can fully relax. Second, towels provide warmth when laid over the body, as the blood pressure lowers during massage and body temperature drops. Third, they provide a feeling of comfort and safety.

Any part of the body that is not being touched should be covered with two or three smaller towels, each one covering a separate part of the body. This method gives you more versatility than if you had one large towel covering the whole body, as you can then reposition the body more easily and it is simpler to change the area you are working on without too much difficulty or upheaval.

As a general rule, the towel is used as a single layer and the top inch or two is either tucked into the edge of any clothing or tucked underneath the rest of the towel to form a

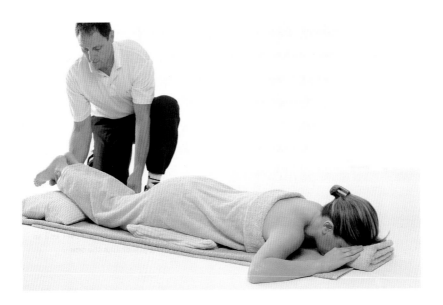

ABOVE **Position the body correctly to boost massage benefits. Place cushions or folded towels under the feet, pelvic area and forehead to provide comfort and protection during the massage.**

definite edge. For large flat areas like backs and abdomens, lay the towel straight over the lower body; for legs and arms it's often easier to use it at an angle along the joint line.

You will need:
- 2 bath towels for general body coverage
- 2 hand towels for specific areas

The towels should be clean and dry. Because some people are allergic to certain washing powders and fabric softeners, it might be a good idea to use a nonbiological detergent. For added luxury, you can warm the towels on a radiator or in a tumble dryer before use.

Working through clothing
If you want to work through clothing, you can use compression and stretch techniques or small circular massage motions, but you will have to avoid sliding or depth work because clothes will cause friction, restrict movement and prevent good contact with the muscle.

The perfect environment
Massage is all about comfort and relaxation, so your surroundings should echo this. Turn down harsh lighting to create a tranquil atmosphere and scent the room with your favourite perfume, incense or aromatherapy oils. Ensure that the person being massaged feels relaxed and comfortable and is not too hot or cold – sometimes being covered with towels can heat the body up too much, so make sure you check how the person feels at regular intervals. Try to make sure you will have peace and quiet, without interruption.

By stimulating all the senses in this way you will magnify the beneficial therapeutic effects of massage on both the body and mind.

You will need:

- Plenty of warm dry towels for covering up massaged areas, keeping the body warm and comforted and preserving modesty.
- Your chosen oil, lotion, cream or talc to provide lubrication, which is especially important on the back because of the large skin area.
- Clean hands and loose, soft clothing so that you feel comfortable and are able to move freely while you massage.
- Soft cushions or pillows to support areas of the body while lying in the optimum positions for being massaged.
- A blanket or thick towel if you are lying on a hard floor.
- A mirror, if required, to check your positioning.
- A glass of water for each person.
- A DO NOT DISTURB sign for the outside of the door if you are likely to be interrupted.

Tips for the masseur:

- Go to the toilet in advance, to make sure you won't have to leave the room mid-massage.
- Turn the lights down low to reduce eyestrain and create an atmosphere. Introduce candles for an alternative and relaxing light source.
- Turn up the heating to ensure the room is warm and draught-free.
- Turn off the phone and any other potential distractions and put on some soft, relaxing, atmospheric music.
- Wash your hands with gently scented soap and warm them.
- Take a moment to focus fully before you start to ease yourself slowly into a calm, centred state of mind. This will ensure that you are ready to give total concentration to the massage.

Tips for the person being massaged:

- Wear comfortable, loose-fitting clothes.
- Remove all bracelets, rings, make-up, contact lenses and glasses.
- Find a comfortable position and be aware of how your body feels.

NOTES

- Test for allergic reactions to creams, oils or lotions and read all the safety guidelines carefully to prevent adverse reactions. If you are worried, the best way to test is to cover a small area of skin on the inside of the arm with the cream 24 hours before you are going to massage and watch for any adverse reactions.
- Check for any contraindications to massage, see pages 12–14, and seek medical advice if you are unsure.
- The person being massaged should allow at least an hour after eating or exercise before having the massage, and avoid stimulants like caffeine in tea, coffee, chocolate and fizzy drinks beforehand.
- Make sure you feel good. You will be in close contact during the time you're giving the massage and infectious or contagious conditions could easily be passed on.
- Cover cuts and scratches on your hands.

Mind-clearing tip

Leave worries and troubles at the door of your massage room and dedicate yourself to the massage. If you find this difficult, use a book to write down all the things that are worrying you and leave it outside the door with your worries. Don't worry about the time you are spending in the massage room either; allow yourself this little treat.

Talk the talk

Take a few minutes to talk to each other about what your expectations are and how you have reacted to treatment in the past. Has the person being massaged ever had a bad or frightening experience? Have they reacted strangely, felt sick, faint or emotional following treatment, or have they suffered allergic reactions to oils, creams or lotions?

Are either of you worried about anything that you should mention? Taking a little time to talk openly will increase the bond between you and give you a platform to clear away worries and troubles before you begin.

BELOW **Massage involves intimate touch, so put each other at ease before the massage begins by talking together.**

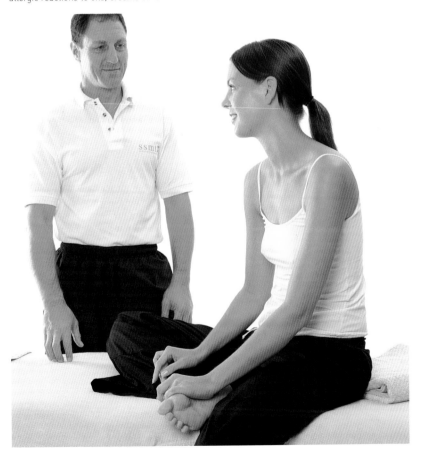

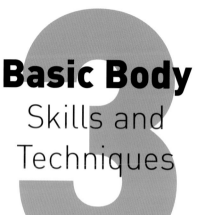

Basic Body
Skills and Techniques

Professional therapists spend years perfecting their techniques, but there are a few tips and essentials you can learn in minutes. Getting to grips with massage is hard work unless you know how to do it right, employing your whole body to soothe away stress and tension and promote healing using strong, fluid strokes.

This chapter shows you how to position yourself and the person you are massaging for ultimate benefit and how to use your body-weight to create controlled, smooth strokes. It shows you techniques like effleurage (stroking), petrissage (kneading) and soft-tissue release stretches, the essential ingredients for a professional-style massage.

The positions in this book are designed for you to pick and mix to target problem areas or to follow a whole series for a thorough, all-over massage. Where no specific starting position is given, continue from the previous technique. Massage is intuitive and understanding the basic techniques will enable you to do what is instinctive.

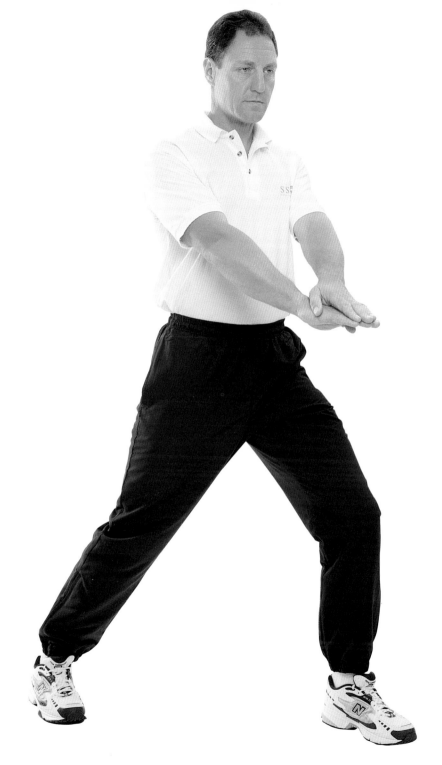

Getting the position right

Professional masseurs have adjustable, transportable couches that help keep the body in a neutral position during massage. To show the perfect massage posture and technique, the procedures explained here assume correct positioning and are described as if a massage bed was being used.

To maximize the benefits of massage, the body must be allowed to totally relax. This means that none of the muscles should be working, the spine and bones should be supported and not stretched, and the head and hips should not be twisted. There are two ways to create a good lying position at home: on the floor and on a bed.

BELOW **The masseur's lower back is straight and his arms are locked.**

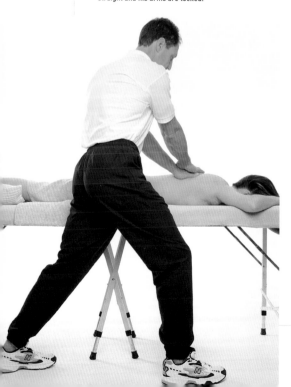

The floor

The floor is usually the best location for a home massage because it is hard and so provides a firm surface for the masseur to push against (a few soft towels or blankets can help to make it more comfortable).

When lying on the back and facing the ceiling (in the 'supine' position), a cushion or pillow should be placed under the knees to reduce pressure on the lower back and a slim towel can be used under the head and lower back for comfort. For lying facing the floor (the 'prone' position), a cushion or pillow should be placed under the hips to raise the lower back and another should be put under the feet so that the knees are bent (see also page 21). The head should be straight, facing the floor and not twisted, and the forehead can either rest on the hands or on a pillow. The arms should be bent at the elbow and resting either side of the head, if they are not forming a platform for the forehead.

Caution: It is most important, for all massage, that the neck is not twisted or cricked. The head should be positioned directly above the spine and the back of the neck lengthened comfortably.

The masseur should kneel (a pillow, towel or cushion can be used) around the body to get into position and use their bodyweight to work the techniques. Sitting cross-legged can be useful when massaging the head and feet.

If the masseur finds kneeling a problem, they may prefer to use a higher surface. If you have a dining-room table, which will take the weight of a body, position the person to be massaged on top of it using the same positions as the floor.

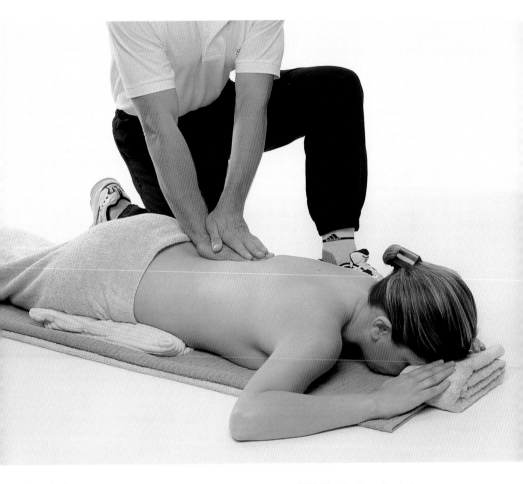

The bed

Beds are not ideal for massage because they are soft, which means the bed rather than the body will move. Positioning is the same as for the floor, but take extra care to ensure that the neck is straight. To massage, come around the side of the bed rather than sitting or kneeling on it. If you have a double bed, massage one side of the body and then move across the bed to massage the other.

ABOVE **If kneeling, the position for the masseur is the same as for standing, with lower arms and back locked.**

Massage is about comfort, both for the person being massaged and the masseur. If there is discomfort or pain, the therapeutic benefits will be lost and you could cause injury or strain. Take the time to create the right atmosphere and find comfortable positions.

Techniques

Massage isn't about having strength in the arms, wrists, hands or thumbs; instead, it is about bodyweight. Much like practitioners of eastern balance arts, such as Tai Chi, masseurs use the weight of their bodies, moving through the hips backwards, forwards and side to side, to create movement. If you watch a professional masseur at work, their back is straight and their shoulders and arms are locked in front of them.

The correct technique is important, not only because it helps you to give the best massage and allows you to control the pressure you are exerting without tiring yourself out, but it also prevents injury and strain, and allows you to relax and enjoy giving a massage as much as receiving one. A masseur who has a good posture does not have to work hard. As long as you are in the right position, the strokes will become smooth, powerful and effortless and the movement instinctive.

For the ultimate comfort of the person being massaged, and to maintain a controlled rhythm throughout the massage techniques, try to avoid removing your hands from the skin while you work. Professional masseurs rarely take their hands off the body, unless it is to add more lotion or oil or to alter their position or the towelling. This constant touch is very important in maintaining and developing a patient-practitioner bond that encourages calm and focuses the massage.

Throughout the massage you should remain aware of your movements. Watch out for any winces, twitches, flinches or movements from the person being massaged that could indicate that you are causing them discomfort or that they are somehow in pain.

Bodyweight balance practise

To get used to using your bodyweight and balance, hold your arms out in front of you, in a circle with your hands together, and sway your hips in order to to move your hands without utilizing your arms. Once you have mastered this, try spreading your feet further apart and, with a smooth lunge, transfer your bodyweight from leg to leg without moving your arms or shoulders. Your back should never bend. If you feel as if you need to bend to exert pressure, bend your knees or move closer to the area being massaged – this should allow you to use the correct technique.

NOTES

- For the comfort of the person being massaged, all techniques require that your nails are short and there are no rough or hard patches on your hands. In addition to this, you should remove all hand and wrist jewellery and watches and have short or rolled-up sleeves.
- The hand of the masseur should always follow the contours of the body, so for some areas, like the forearms and shins, it is sometimes better to use the hand sideways so it fits over the natural curve of the skin.
- If your thumbs, hands, wrists or arms start to ache, it is likely that you are using them directly, instead of using your bodyweight, to exert pressure. To avoid this problem, practise moving around on your feet by using your hips to balance and keeping your shoulders and arms in position without bending them. If you use your weight instead of your muscles, the massage won't feel like such hard work.

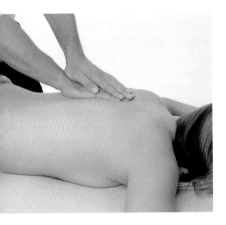

▲ Technique 1: Effleurage

Also known as stroking, effleurage is good for clearing blood, lymph and body fluids, warming up the muscle group and boosting circulation. Using the palm, side or heel of the hand push into the skin and tissues beneath. It can be one- or two-handed and should start slowly, building to the middle of the stroke and tapering off at the end. The strokes should be hard enough to cause some redness and warmth in the skin. Typically, you would start a massage with this, to warm the area for deeper work.

1 Place one hand flat, palm down, with the fingers pointing forwards.
2 Place the other hand over the palm.
3 Lock wrists and elbows.
4 Use your bodyweight to move yourself slowly forwards.
5 DO NOT bend your back – movement should come from knees and hips.
6 Take three or four small strokes and then follow with a single long stroke.
7 For large areas, use a lunge technique. Stand with one leg in front and then transfer your weight to move forwards.

▼ Technique 2: Deep effleurage

This technique is similar to effleurage except that you use the thumbs, which allows a deeper penetration of the body tissues. The basic technique is the same, using the transfer of bodyweight to exert pressure. You are looking for a slight wave of skin in front of the thumb and reddening of the skin in the areas you have worked on; the massage should feel deep, but not painful.

1 Place one hand palm down on the area with the thumb flat.
2 Place the other thumb over the first. For small areas like the arms use a thumb on top, and for large areas like the back and thighs you can place the heel of the hand over the thumb.
3 Lock thumbs, wrists and elbows.
4 Exert pressure through thumbs and, using bodyweight, work away from you.

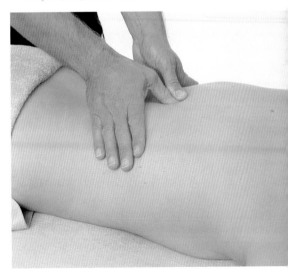

▼ Technique 3: Petrissage

Petrissage employs both hands working in opposite directions to free up problem areas, boost circulation and work deep into muscles (see page 93 for a close-up of the technique).

1 Place both hands palm down, side by side, and lock the thumbs, wrists and elbows in position.
2 Roll your hips right and forwards so that your right thumb moves forward.
3 At the same time, bring the fingers of the left hand back so that they meet and glide over the right thumb.
4 Roll your hips to the left so that your left thumb moves forwards and bring your right fingers back to meet it.
5 Keep both palms on the skin as pivots.
6 Continue to work the rhythm, bringing thumb and fingers together alternately as your hips roll to move your weight.
7 Your shoulders should move with your hips, and should not be still.

▼ Technique 4: Cam and spindle

Cam and spindle is a deep muscle technique for releasing tension and working into the tissues. It employs the knuckles of one hand (the 'cam') and the palm of the other (the 'spindle') working together to penetrate deeply.

1 Make a fist with one hand then join the hands by inserting the thumb of the other hand into the clenched fingers of the fist.
2 Lock your wrists and elbows and, using the outstretched hand (spindle) as a guide and the fist (cam) to massage the muscle, work in small straight motions away from you.
3 To increase pressure, tighten the fist around the thumb and to decrease pressure, loosen the fist.

tip Never cam and spindle over bone; it is a deep technique that could cause harm.

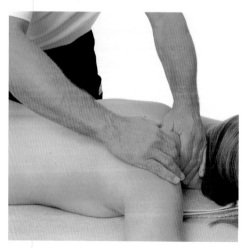

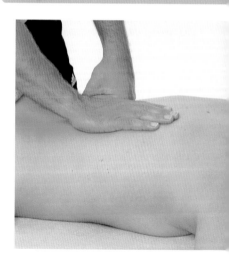

Basic body skills and techniques

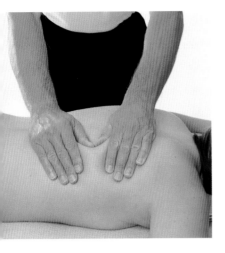

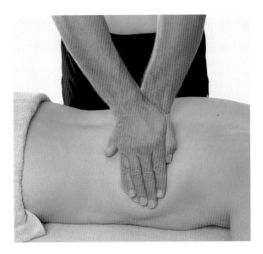

▲ Technique 5: Dermal lifting

Dermal lifting helps boost circulation into the skin by working the deep layers as well as the surface. This increases blood flow and stimulates growth and healing.

1 Place both hands palm down on the skin, forming a triangle between your thumbs and fingers.
2 Move your thumbs forward, using your bodyweight, so that they push into the triangle towards the fingers, raising a wave of skin in front of them.
3 Continue moving the thumbs forwards until a triangle of skin is trapped between the thumb and fingers, then release and work the next area.
4 Work the rhythm by rocking back and forth on your hips to create a controlled movement.

▲ Technique 6: Compression

Compression is one of the most simple massage techniques and also one of the most effective. It stimulates blood and lymph flow and releases tension.

1 Place one hand on the skin with your fingers raised and the heel of the hand prepared to press down.
2 Place the other hand on top of the heel of the contact hand, keeping the fingers relaxed.
3 Using your bodyweight, press down on the area for at least three seconds, and then slowly release the pressure.
4 Move to a new area and create a rhythm by rocking on your hips to produce and release pressure.
5 You should not compress the same area twice.

Techniques

tip Locking the arms does not mean that they have to be straight; they should be firm but relaxed, and you should move them by using only your bodyweight and not your muscles.

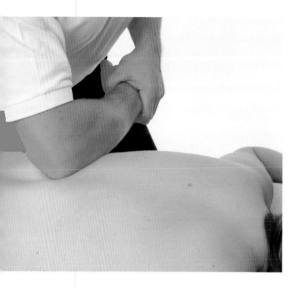

▲ Using other parts of your body

In some cases the hands and thumbs might not be strong enough to exert effective pressure. In this case elbows can be used for deeper penetration.

1　Stand with your elbow by your side, directly under your shoulder.
2　Place one leg in front of you and transfer your weight forward, keeping your elbow under your shoulder.
3　Be aware that although the elbow gives you deeper penetration you lose sensation; it is important to keep going back to using your hands so you can feel the muscle as well.
4　You can also use the forearm, which exerts a broader and therefore more superficial pressure. Do this in the same way as the elbow, placing your whole forearm on the area to be massaged and holding the wrist with the other hand to stabilize the posture.

▼ Technique 7: STR (Soft Tissue Release)

STR is a specialized technique used for stretching the muscle fibres using the thumb to exert pressure on the muscle and the other hand to move the muscle into a stretch.

1　Unload the muscle – here the arm is bent at the elbow and the hand supported so the muscle isn't working.
2　Lock the thumb into the muscle – press the flat of the thumb directly into the muscle at the centre of the arm. Use the thumb to stretch the relaxed muscle upwards. Press upwards by moving the thumb 1 cm (½ in) towards

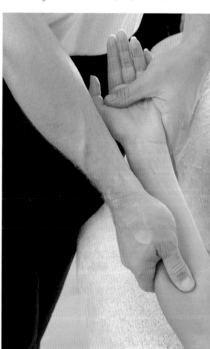

the top of the muscle. This action will stretch the muscle fibres underneath.

3   Load the stretch – keeping the thumb in position, slowly move the muscle into a stretch by moving the wrist downwards to straighten the elbow. Where the thumb is exerting pressure, it will stretch the muscle beneath it.

4   Work into the rest of the muscle – repeat the unload-lock-load-stretch process three or four times, making sure that you work on different areas of the muscle while covering the entire length of the arm, or whatever area you happen to be massaging.

5   Do not work on the same area twice.

▼ Technique 8: Stretch and draw

Stretch and draw combines the long strokes of effleurage with a stretching technique. It is performed towards you for greater control.

1   Position yourself on one side of the body, with your hands on the other side.

2   Form a loose hook with the fingers.

3   Bending your knees, bring your weight backwards, draw the hands slowly towards you, stretching the skin and tissues underneath it.

4   As you come to the end of the stretch and draw stroke, ease off – under control – by straightening your knees.

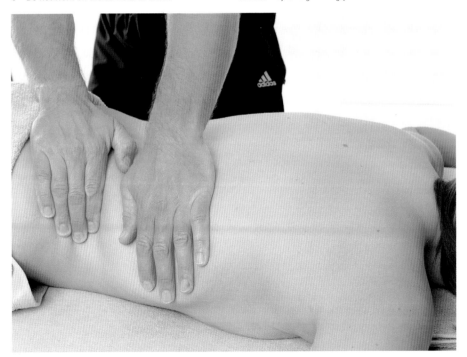

Back, Neck and
Shoulder Massage

Of all the areas of the body, the head, neck and shoulders are the most prone to stress. Everyday stress and activity makes muscles tighten and eyes, jaws and necks tense up. Massage helps ease away tension and stress, boosting circulation and flexibility and preventing stiffness, pain, injury and trauma.

This series of massages shows you how to give a total back, neck and shoulder massage to one side of the body. For an entire session, complete all the massages on both sides of the body, either by exposing the whole back and performing a page at a time on both sides or by concentrating on one side at a time.

The back, neck and shoulders massage series should take about 40 minutes if you follow the book, but you can vary or personalize the massage by spending longer or less time on certain techniques or even skipping some altogether. You should always finish with the back relaxation stroke, which will complete the massage.

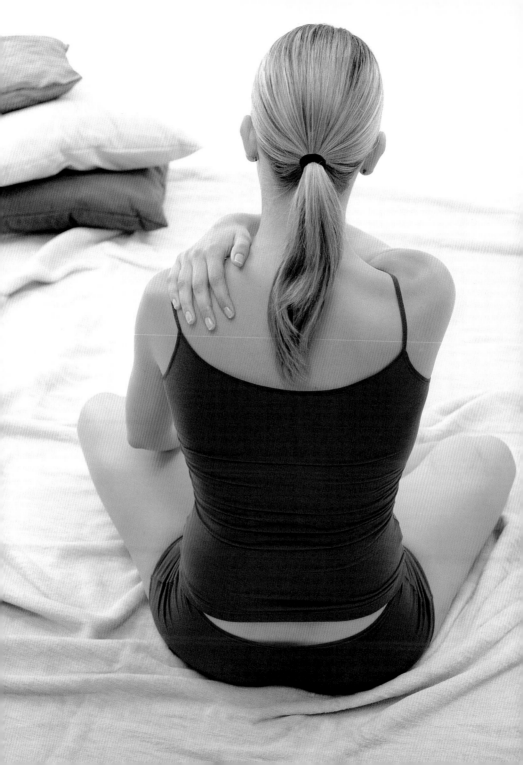

Basic anatomy

In order to understand how best to massage the back, neck and shoulders, the masseur needs to have a basic knowledge of anatomy. The bones and muscles will be discussed here but, it is important to remember that no single thing in our body works in isolation.

Bones of the back, neck and shoulders

The bones of the back, neck and shoulders are balanced on top of the pelvic girdle, a plate of bone at hip level that sits on top of the legs to provide balance and support to the upper body. The spine is composed of bones called vertebrae that sit on top of each other and have a hole running down the middle through which travels the spinal cord and blood supply that provides feeling, nerve control, blood and lymph to the lower limbs.

The top vertebra, which is attached to the occiput bone at the base of the skull, is the only spinal joint that does not move. Together, the vertebrae form a loose S-shape that curves in towards the stomach and lower back, out at the middle back and slightly in again at the neck. When the spine is in this position, the 'neutral position', it supports its own weight with no stress, strain or tiring muscle activity. We work in and towards this position during massage.

The balance of the body comes from the legs. Visualize the bones by working upwards from the pelvic girdle:

Pelvic girdle – A bony plate running across the width of the body to provide strength, balance and support to the upper body.
Sacroiliac joint – Five vertebrae that fuse during puberty to form a strength-bearing joint at the bottom of the spine.

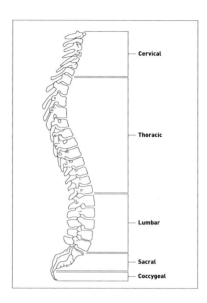

ABOVE **There are 24 moving vertebrae in the spine, with soft tissue discs between each one.**

Lumbar spine – The five largest vertebrae making up the lower part of the back. They form a natural curve, with the apex towards the front of the body (a lordotic curve).
Thoracic spine – The twelve vertebrae, to which the ribs attach, forming the central part of the back. They form slight curve with the apex away from the front of the body (a kyphotic curve).
Cervical spine – The seven small vertebrae of the upper part of the back that form a lordotic curve. The top two form a joint on which the head can pivot.
Clavicles – Two collarbones, one on each side, give stability and movement to the shoulders and attach them to the fixed, stable breastbone (sternum).
Scapulas – The two triangular shoulder blades that attach to and support the arm.

The labels on the figure read:
- Cervical
- Thoracic
- Lumbar
- Sacral
- Coccygeal

Between the vertebrae are gel-filled discs that allow the bones to move and provide a shock-absorbing casing for the spinal cord. These intervertebral discs account for one-third of the spine length and increase its weight-bearing capacity. It is important not to perform massage techniques directly on the spine as this could cause injury. The vertebrae are used as a guide only to massage the muscles at the sides of the spine. Special care must be taken with the neck vertebrae, which are more mobile and prone to injury.

Muscles of the back, neck and shoulders

The muscles of the back, neck and shoulders perform three tasks – stability to the trunk and upper body through the spine, movement of the head and neck on top of the spine and movement and rotation of the arms.

The main vertical muscles of the back are the paraspinal muscles, which run up either side of the spine to provide support. Two trapezius muscles run across the top of the back to stabilize the shoulder blades. The main muscles in the centre of the back are the latissimus dorsi, which start at the centre of the spine and wrap around and up the back to finish at the sides of the ribcage. Around the sides of the lower back, oblique muscles keep the trunk and abdomen upright. At the lower end of the spine, the large gluteal muscles run down over the bottom and around the hip. These stabilize the pelvic girdle to provide a balancing point for the whole upper body.

Blood and nerve supply

The major blood vessels serving the back, neck and shoulders run down the spine. The carotid artery runs up the side of the neck, taking oxygenated blood to the neck, head and brain, and the jugular vein returns the blood to the heart. The neck and back are the channels for the body's nervous system as the spinal cord runs through the spine.

BELOW **The major muscles of the back give support and stability to the body.**

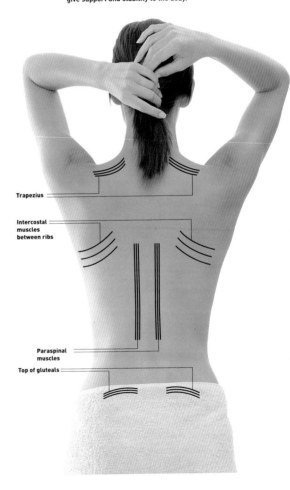

Trapezius

Intercostal
muscles
between ribs

Paraspinal
muscles

Top of gluteals

BEFORE YOU BEGIN this section, make sure that the person to be massaged is lying supine – on their back, facing the ceiling. In each technique where no specific position is given, the person should be lying in the same starting position as described in the previous technique.

tip Remember to use your bodyweight for exerting pressure. If you are finding it difficult to do this, or you can't remember what it feels like, run through the bodyweight balance practise techniques on page 28.

▼ Clavicular effleurage

To ease tension and soreness in the front of the shoulders.

1   Face the left shoulder of the person being massaged.
2   Place the first two fingers of the right hand in the centre of the upper chest just under the collarbone (or clavicle), with fingers facing the right shoulder.
3   Place the first two fingers of the left hand on top and move your bodyweight forwards to move the fingers along underneath the bone, finishing at the shoulder.
4   Rock backwards, dragging the fingers lightly over the skin surface, and repeat several times on both sides.

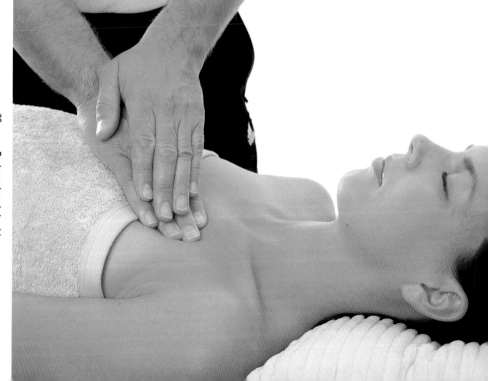

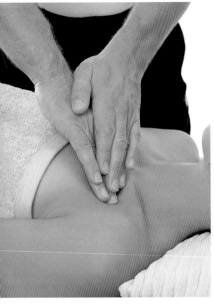

▼ Sternal and clavicular chest stretch

To stretch out the chest muscles, which may be tight due to stress or bad posture.

1 Stand to the right facing the shoulder.
2 Pick up the right arm by the wrist so it is level with the shoulder, pointing towards the ceiling, and support it.
3 Place the heel of your right hand into the side of the chest and push gently while you bring the arm down. Maintain pressure until the elbow is level with the shoulder.
4 To stretch through the chest, pick up the arm by the wrist with both hands. Step backwards and let the arm drop until it is level with the shoulder.

▲ Sternal effleurage

To ease tension in the chest.

1 Place four fingers of the right hand as before, with the left hand positioned palm down over the fingers.
2 Starting centrally, work all four fingers along the line of the collarbone, lightening the stroke towards the end and then back lightly over the skin.
3 Repeat several times on both sides.

Deep effleurage of the chest (optional)

1 Position as above, but this time use the thumb of the right hand, covered by the thumb of the left. Perform a deep stroke across the chest from the centre to the side of the shoulder.

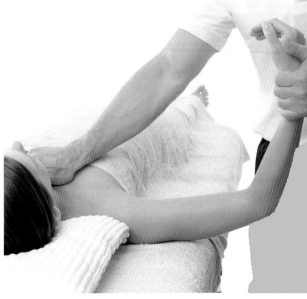

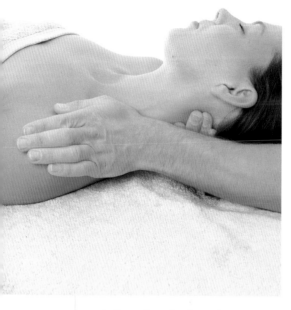

▼ Transverse neck effleurage

To work deeper and further into the neck muscles.

1 Position yourself as previously but this time, instead of using the heel of your hand to stroke down the neck, use your thumb to stroke in a downward motion from the front of the neck to the back.
2 Start with your thumb at the base of the ear and draw the thumb down over the side of the neck, working your way down the neck in three or four parallel strokes.

▲ One-handed neck effleurage

To drive out tension from stress and bad posture, from the sides of the neck.

1 Position yourself behind the head, facing down the body.
2 Cup your right hand under the neck, cradling the neck in your hand and allowing the head to rest on it.
3 Bring the fingers of your right hand gently towards you, bringing the right ear down towards the right shoulder and exposing the left side of the neck.
4 Place the heel of the left hand on the top of the neck and slide it away from you, towards the top of the shoulder. Remember to keep the right hand very still as it supports the head.

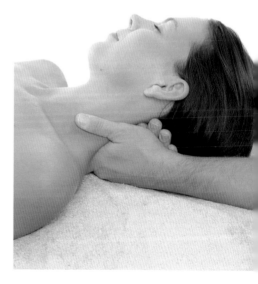

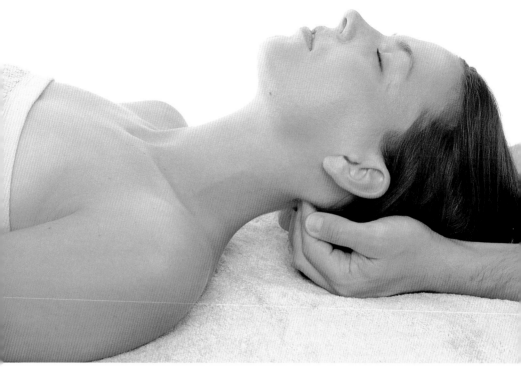

▲ Occiput pressure release

To relieve pressure, tension and stress
from the muscles at the base of the
skull, which can cause headaches, neck
and back pain.

1 Position yourself behind the head
   facing down the body as before.
2 Cup both hands under the head and
   cradle the weight in your hands. Have
   your fingers at the base of the skull,
   under the ridge of bone (the occiput).
3 With the ends of your fingers, make
   small gentle circular movements
   around the base of the skull, being
   careful not to apply too much pressure.
4 Work your way around the whole
   bottom of the skull from the centre to
   the base of each ear and back again.

BEFORE THE NEXT technique, direct the
person being massaged to turn onto their
stomach so the massage can be performed
with the body lying prone (facing the floor).

Occiput deep effleurage

To work further into the occiput.

1 Face the left side of the neck. The
   head and the neck should be in line.
2 Place your right thumb in the centre
   of the neck at the occiput.
3 Using the rest of your right hand to
   stabilize the thumb, stroke down along
   the ridge of bone towards the base
   of the ear. Take care not to press too
   hard, if the person feels any pain, or
   altered sensation in or around the
   eyes, you must stop immediately.

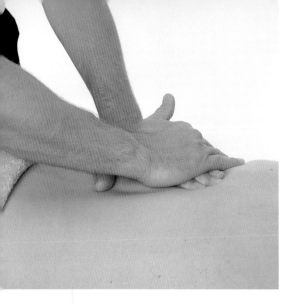

▲ Spinal four-fingered effleurage

To relax and release tension in the spine before starting deeper techniques.

1 Position yourself at the middle of the left side facing the opposite shoulder.
2 Place the first two fingers of your left hand beside the spine on the side closest to you, on the ridge of muscle that runs up beside the spine (the paraspinal muscles).
3 Cover these fingers with the palm of the other hand and work up the paraspinals to halfway. While doing this, you should be pressing hard enough to create a slight wave of skin in front of your fingers.
4 In this way work your way up the back in three overlapping strokes: make one stroke from the bottom to halfway, then one from a quarter of the way to three-quarters, then one from halfway to the top, tapering the stroke on the shoulder in a controlled way without allowing the stroke to fall off the shoulder.

▼ Spinal thumb effleurage

To work deeper into the spine muscles.

1 Place your right hand on the bottom of the spine with the thumb and fingers at right angles. Lay the thumb beside, but not on, the spine on the side nearest to you, and the fingers pointing up the spine.
2 Place the left thumb on top of the right thumb and work your way up the back, exerting enough pressure to form a slight wave of skin in front of your thumb.
3 Instead of working up the back in one long stroke, which could force you to bend your back, work in three or four shorter strokes to cover the whole length, with overlaps between strokes. To move forwards, perform a lunging motion with your left leg and shift your bodyweight smoothly onto it.
4 Remember to keep your hands lightly on the skin between strokes to maximize relaxation potential.

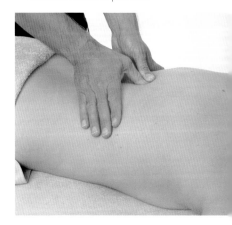

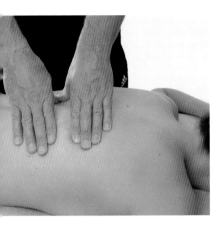

▲ Transverse thumb effleurage away from the spine

To stretch the spinal muscles away from the spine and reduce tension caused by bad posture.

1   Face the lower back.
2   Starting at the bottom of the back, place your right thumb on the side of the spine nearest to you (beside the spine, not on top of it).
3   Place your left thumb on top of the right and stroke towards you, finishing in a controlled way before your thumbs drop off the side.
4   Place your thumbs at the side of the spine about 5 cm (2 in) further up and repeat.
5   Work your way up the spine in this way, moving up every 5 cm (2 in) or so after each separate stroke, to finish at the shoulder blade.

tip If your thumbs begin to get tired while performing the effleurage techniques here, make sure that they are locked in position with no bending of the hand or wrist. Remember to use your bodyweight for exerting pressure.

▼ Circular shoulder effleurage

To reduce pressure and tension which can build up in the shoulders due to stress and bad posture.

1   Face the left shoulder.
2   Put your right hand palm down, fingers towards the head, next to the spine on the side furthest from you.
3   Raise your fingers slightly and stroke the heel of the hand up the spine until it reaches the neck.
4   Move the hand sideways on to the top of the shoulder in a circular motion and finish the stroke with control, just before the heel of your hand falls off.

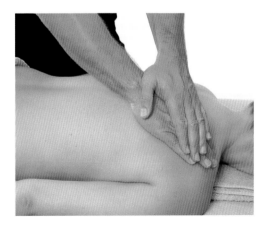

▼ Spine to shoulder blade effleurage

To release tension in the shoulder blades.

1 Face the left shoulder.
2 Reach over and place the flat of your right thumb at the nape of the neck on the opposite side of the body and cover it with the left forefingers.
3 Using the fingers of your right hand as a guide, make a straight stroke down from the base of the neck towards the top of the shoulder.
4 Move your thumb to the starting point, shift down 2.5 cm (1 in) and make a second stroke parallel to the first.
5 Repeat the downward movement between strokes and finish halfway down the shoulder.

Neck to shoulder blade effleurage

To work deep into the postural muscles at the side of the neck to reduce tension and increase movement.

1 Position yourself at the left of the neck with your body inclined towards the feet of the person being massaged.
2 Reach over and position your right thumb just below the hairline on the right side.
3 Cover your right thumb with your left thumb and make a gentle stroke down the neck towards the top of the shoulder, ending the stroke where the shoulder bone meets the arm.

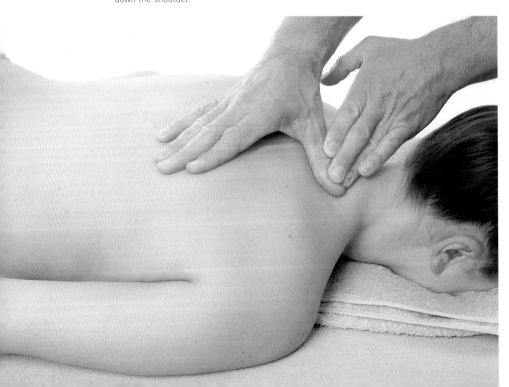

▼ Shoulder petrissage

**To work deep into the postural muscles
at the top of the neck to reduce tension
and work away muscle knots.**

1   Position yourself at the left of the
    neck with your body inclined towards
    the head.
2   Reach over to the right side of the
    neck and place your left hand on
    the side of the neck and your right
    hand at the bottom of the neck,
    where it curves into the shoulder.
3   Petrissage this area, starting very
    gently, bringing the left thumb to
    the right fingers and the right thumb
    to the left fingers.

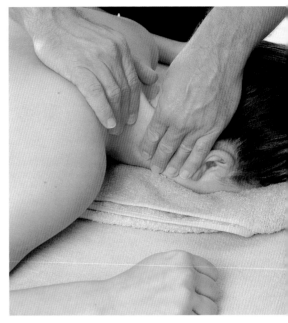

▲ Neck petrissage

**To work deeply across the muscles
of the neck.**

1   Position yourself to the left side of
    the neck.
2   Reach over the body and place both
    hands gently on the opposite side of
    the neck.
3   Using gentle movements, bring
    alternate fingers and thumbs together
    to petrissage the muscles at the side
    of the neck. Take care not to exert too
    much pressure in this area. If in
    doubt, ease off.

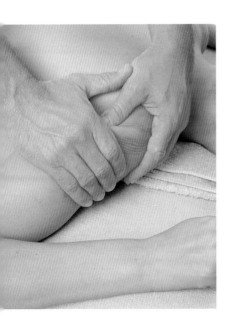

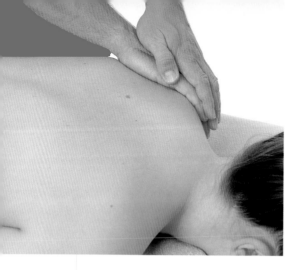

▼ Spine to central shoulder blade effleurage

This technique and the next one – the lower shoulder blade effleurage – work deep to increase postural flexibility.

1 Gently place the left arm by the side of the body, then position yourself on that side facing the head.
3 Use your whole hand to grasp the fleshy circular area that lies on top of the shoulder and raise until you see the shoulder blade lift up off the back. Remember not to bend your back.
4 Hold this position with your left hand and use the flattened fingers of your right hand to stroke in and around the edges of the shoulder blade. The thumb of your right hand should trail after the fingers around the contours of the shoulder blade.

▲ Neck stretch and draw

To pull the shoulders away from the neck to reduce bunched up muscle tension in this area.

1 Position yourself at the left side of the ribs with your body facing the head.
2 Place your right hand on top of the shoulder so that your fingers disappear over the edge at the front of the shoulder, towards the arm.
3 Form a loose hook with your fingers so that you feel the shoulder underneath them.
4 Lock the fingers in place and gently draw the hand back, over and across the skin, using your bodyweight to perform the movement. Keep all parts of your hand in contact with the skin at all times, gently releasing the hooking of your fingers as your hand moves backwards.
5 End the stroke when your hand lies flat on top of the shoulder and the fingers are no longer hooked.

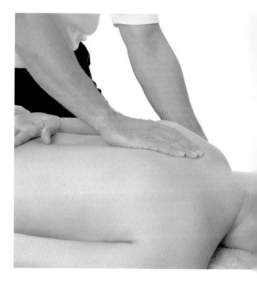

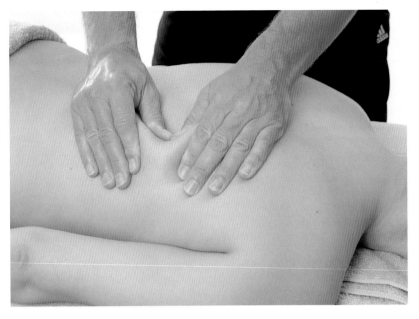

Lower shoulder blade effleurage

1 Face the right ribcage.
2 Reach over to the other side of the body with your left palm and cover it with your right, positioning the two palms face down at the bottom of the shoulder blade just the other side of the spine. Do not touch the spine.
3 Following the line of the ribs, stroke along the bottom of the shoulder blade, finishing the stroke as it tapers off the side of the body.

▲ Dermal lifting of the middle back

To boost circulation to the thick skin at the centre of the back in order to stimulate nerves and boost skin health.

1 Position yourself at the left side facing the middle of the back.
2 Place the flats of both thumbs on the opposite side of the body, off the spine.
3 Using the thumbs and first fingers of both hands, alternately pick up and drop sections of skin, working smoothly to create a lifting rhythm, taking care not to pinch the skin.
4 The movement should feel fluid and smooth, not jerky or painful. Work your way down from the spine towards the side of the body and sideways towards the lower back.

▼ Dermal rolling of the middle back

To work into the deep levels of the skin to boost circulation.

1 Make sure you have lubricated the skin as dermal rolling is a high-friction technique.
2 Place both hands on the opposite side of the body with the thumbs placed flat along the ridge of muscle that runs next to the spine and the fingers of both hands forming a triangle that points towards the side of the body.
3 Lift and roll the skin in this triangle, working side to side and forwards and backwards to cover the whole middle back area down to the lower back and up to the shoulder blade.

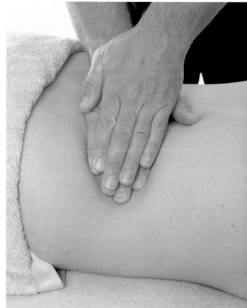

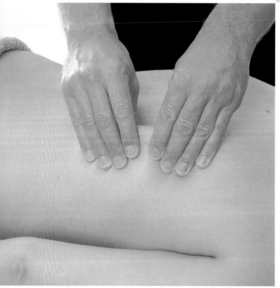

▲ Lower back effleurage

To ease pain and tension in the lower back and prepare for deeper massage.

1 Face the left lower back.
2 Place your right palm down on the V-shaped bone at the bottom of the spine, with the heel of your hand against the V and your fingers pointing away, towards the opposite side.
3 Place your left palm down, so that it covers your right hand.
4 Slowly start to press down with the palms and stroke away from you towards the top of the hip, easing off when you reach the hip.
5 At the end of the stroke, drag the fingers lightly across the skin to the starting position and repeat.

▼ Deep thumb lower back effleurage

To work deep into the lower back.

1 Face the left lower back.
2 On the side closest to you, place your right thumb just in front of the V at the bottom of the spine, with the fingers at right angles to the thumb.
3 Place your left thumb over the right. Stroke gently down towards the top of the hip (towards you), releasing the pressure to finish the stroke smoothly and returning the hand to the starting position. Maintain a light pressure on the skin so that you don't break contact.
4 Repeat several times, applying slightly more pressure each time for deeper and deeper effleurage.

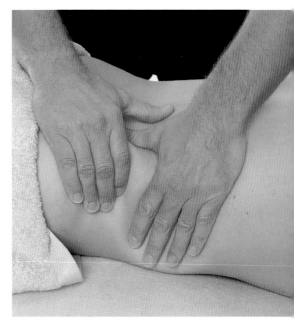

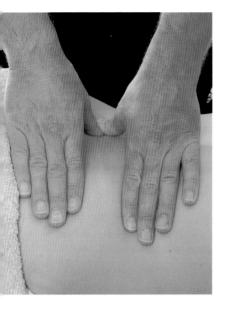

▲ Lower back petrissage

To boost circulation in the skin and muscles of the lower back.

1 Face the left middle back.
2 Bend your knees and place both hands on the other side of the spine with fingers facing away from you, down towards the side of the body.
3 Petrissage, bringing alternate thumbs and fingers together using your bodyweight to create a rhythm.
4 Work your way from the spine down towards the side of the body. Then move down towards the bottom of the back and repeat the movement.

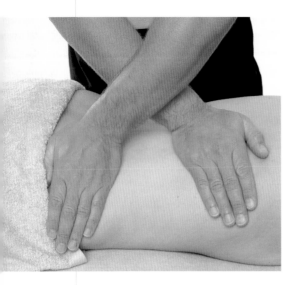

▼ Transverse draw around hip

To work away tension and knots in the muscles that lie at the side and centre of the lower back.

1 Bend your knees, straighten your back and rock forwards to allow you to lean over the body without stretching or bending your back.
2 Place the left palm on the side of the hip, with the fingers facing towards the front of the hip and make a loose hook with the ends of the fingers. You should be able to feel the front of the hip in your fingers.
3 Place the right hand on top of the left hand for strength and stability.
4 Lock the arms and wrists in position. This is very important for stretch and draw techniques because they involve

▲ Lower back stretch (with crossed arms)

To stretch the muscles of the lower back and release tension from bad posture.

1 Face the left lower back.
2 Cross your arms over each other and place the hands palm down in the middle of the lower back. The little fingers should be together and the heels of the hands next to, but not touching, the spine.
3 Push your bodyweight down and, as you do so, allow the hands to spread apart, stretching the skin beneath.
4 Continue the stretch as far as you feel comfortable with crossed hands, or until the lower hand reaches the bottom of the back. Then straighten your knees and lift up your body (to reduce the pressure going through your hands) to end the stretch in a controlled manner.

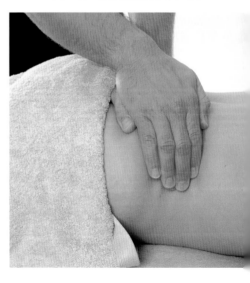

quite a lot of bodyweight transfer, which can cause back problems if not performed correctly.

5   Rock backwards and upwards, straightening your knees and controlling your bodyweight transfer, and draw the hands around the hip towards the V-shaped bone at the bottom of the spine. Gradually loosen the hooked fingers as they travel around to the centre so that by the time the heel of your hand arrives at the bottom of the spine, the palm is flat. Repeat once more.

6   Take a step up towards the head and repeat the draw, this time finishing at the base of the ribs instead of at the bottom of the spine.

▶Cam and spindle of lower back

1   Position yourself on the left side of the lower back.

2   Place your right palm down over the spine, with the thumb at right angles facing the head.

3   Make a fist with your left hand around the thumb of the right hand without moving it.

4   The left hand should not come into contact with bone at all. Be very careful; this is a deep massage technique that could cause problems if performed incorrectly.

5   Step forwards with your right leg and lunge forwards onto it very slowly, beginning to work the cam and spindle away from you. Use the right hand as a guide and the left hand to produce a deep massage. Release the pressure as your hands taper off the back.

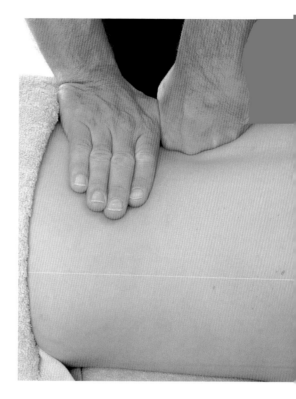

6   **Variation:** For a deep massage of the paraspinal muscles, you can perform a cam and spindle technique working your fist up the muscles at the side of the spine, from the bottom of the back towards the shoulders. Take care to avoid applying pressure on the spine – deep techniques are for massaging muscles only.

▼ Transverse draw of gluteals

To ease tension and knots in the muscles at the top of the buttocks.

1 Face the left lower back. You will need to work in a straight line over the top of the buttocks, rather than arcing over the lower back as in the transverse draw on pages 50–51.
2 Bend your knees, straighten your back and rock forwards to allow you to lean over the body without stretching or bending your back.
3 Place the right palm on top of the hip with the fingers facing towards the front and make a loose hook with the ends of the fingers.

4 Place your left hand on top of your right hand for extra strength and stability. Lock the arms and wrists in position.
5 Rock backwards and upwards, straightening your knees and controlling your bodyweight transfer, and draw your hands around from the hip and over the top of the buttocks towards the V-shaped bone at the bottom of the spine, gradually loosening the hooked fingers as your hands travel around to the centre of the buttocks.
6 By the time the heel of your hand arrives at the bottom of the spine, the palm should be flat over the bottom of the back. Repeat once more to complete.

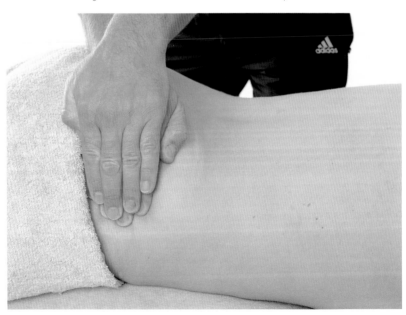

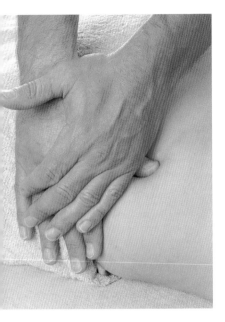

▲ Single thumb stroke of top of buttocks

To work deeper into the sitting and standing muscles.

1   Bend your knees, straighten your back and rock forwards to allow you to lean over the body.
2   Place your right thumb on the V at the bottom of the spine with the fingers pointing towards the side of the body.
3   Cover the right thumb with the heel of the left hand and make a deep stroke over the top of the buttocks, towards the hipbone.
4   Remember to keep your back straight as you finish the stroke on the side of the buttock, by the hip, and draw it back, keeping in soft contact with the skin. Repeat once more.

▼ Cam and spindle of top of buttocks

To reach into the deepest levels of the soft tissues that underpin the lower back.

1   Bend your knees, straighten your back and rock forwards to allow you to lean over the body without bending.
2   Place your left hand on the opposite side of the base of the spine so that the thumb points towards the feet and fingers point towards the side.
3   Make a fist with your right hand around the left thumb, so the knuckles of the right hand sit at the top of the buttock.
4   Using small, deep strokes, work your way around the top of the buttocks towards the side of the hip.

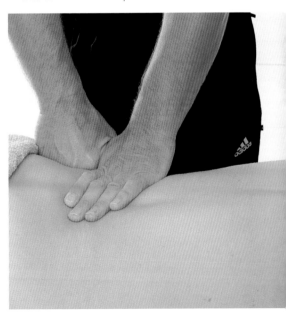

▶ Complete back relaxation stroke

To finish off the back, neck and shoulder massage by using relaxing strokes to ease away any remaining residual tension in the muscles and soft tissues. It also encourages regeneration and healing within the skin, as well as using a caring touch to boost self-esteem and inner peacefulness.

These steps should be performed as one big movement down the spine and back up again. However, to extend the feeling of relaxation, the steps can be performed separately as a four-step process that can be followed with the complete stroke.

1   Position yourself at the head of the person being massaged, looking directly down the body. Because this is a warming-down relaxation process, a lighter touch should be used than for other massages.
2   This stroke requires a lot of body movement, so before you start, position yourself in a lunge position so that you can shift further backwards and forwards without strain or stretching. (For a floor alternative, try kneeling on one knee and placing the other foot on the ground. This allows you to move forwards and backwards smoothly.)
3   Place your hands either side of the spine at the base of the neck, just on top of the shoulders, raise up the fingers of both hands and make a

single stroke straight down the spine with the palms of the hands, finishing at the bottom of the spine with the heels of the hands touching the top of the buttocks.
4   When the heels of your hands touch the top of the buttocks, twist the hands slightly so that the fingers face inwards and the palms face out towards the hips.
5   Push your hands out towards the hips, with the palms leading and the fingers following, in a curved motion that reaches down the sides of the back at lower back level.
6   Using your palms to lead the fingers, bring the hands up the back and closer together so that they lightly touch each other at the level of the shoulder blades. Remember to use your own bodyweight to bring the stroke back towards you, rather than the muscles of your hands, arms or shoulders.
7   Using the palms to lead the hands away from each other, bring the stroke out over the shoulder blades and trace a small circle around the top of the shoulder, bringing your palms on top of the shoulder.
8   When your palms reach the top of the shoulder, shift your bodyweight again to go forwards and move the palms towards the outside of the ribcage at chest level, fingers forward. Finish the stroke by lightly bringing your hands off the skin.
9   Repeat the stroke several times, as required.

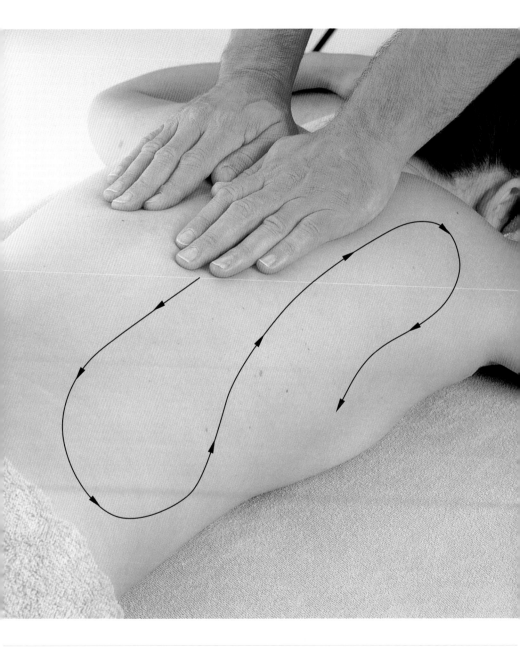

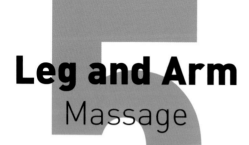

Leg and Arm
Massage

This chapter will show you how to give a total
arm and leg massage to treat tired limbs, boost
the flow of blood and lymph back to the heart
and encourage the renewal and rejuvenation of cells.
Unlike the back, neck and shoulders, where the main benefit of
massage is to relax tension held in postural muscles and drive away
muscle fatigue and tiredness, massage in the arms and legs is also
useful for helping the circulatory and lymphatic drainage systems.

The total arm and leg massage should take about 40 minutes,
but you can pick and choose techniques to highlight specific areas
or just concentrate on the upper or lower limbs, which take about
20 minutes each to do. You should start with a clearance technique
(see pages 60–61) and finish with limb vibrations (see pages 70–71
and 83) to relax any residual tightness in muscles. Because the
muscles of the legs and arms lie near the surface you can develop
your own intuitive touch by responding to what your hands encounter.

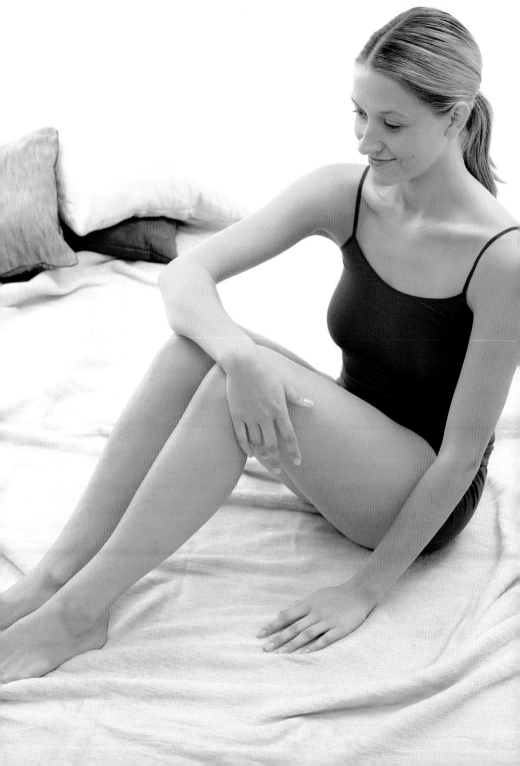

Basic anatomy

The limbs undergo different stresses and strains to the rest of the body because they are the most flexible. Thick arteries and veins run to and from the heart to our limbs. A complex system of nerves control feeling, muscles give a wide range of movement in all directions, and sensory receptors in the skin respond to minute fluctuations in touch, temperature and positioning. Massage benefits all these systems and is particularly good for boosting fluid drainage and return of blood from the extremities.

The difference between the arms and legs is that the legs are weight bearing and the arms are not. Because of this, the muscles in the arms and legs have slightly different qualities – the legs are built for strength and balance while the arms are designed for controlled and complicated movements.

The arms
Bones

The arm hangs from the shoulder joint, a ball and socket that is held in place by the muscles of the shoulder. The long bone at the top of the arm, which runs from shoulder to elbow, is called the humerus. At the elbow joint, this is attached to the two bones of the forearm, the ulna and radius. At the wrist, the ulna and radius attach, via a network of ligaments and tendons, to the hand bones.

Muscles

Each of the major muscle groups contains several individual muscles that work together to take the arm through its whole range of movement. Massage of the arm not only prevents blockage in the muscles but also reduces swelling, decreases tension and boosts circulation in and around tendons

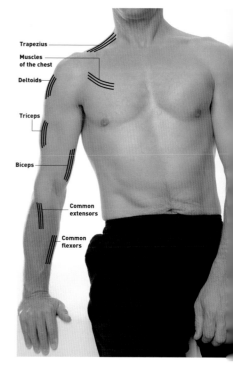

ABOVE **The major muscles of the arm benefit from massage to keep them supple and at a full range of movement.**

to increase efficiency, power and flexibility. Several major muscle groups of the arm, arranged in opposing (antagonistic) pairs, are responsible for movement:

- The muscles in the chest contract to bring the shoulder forwards.
- The trapezius muscles that run from the back of the shoulder across the back, contract to bring the shoulder backwards.
- The deltoid muscles on top of the shoulder, and curving over the arm, contract to bring the arm upwards.

- The muscles in the underarm contract to bring the arm down.
- The biceps at the front of the top arm contract to bend the elbow.
- The triceps, which are opposite the biceps at the back of the arm, contract to straighten the arm.
- The common extensors, on top of the forearm, contract to raise the fingers of the hand and extend the wrist.
- The common flexors, at the bottom of the forearm, flex the wrist bring the fingers up.

Blood and nerve supply

The major artery of the arm, the brachial artery, runs through the shoulder and down to the elbow where it branches into two through the lower arm. The veins follow the same path, in the opposite direction. The brachial nerve runs through the shoulder into the top of the arm and the medial and ulnar nerves supply the whole arm with motor control and sensation.

The legs

Our legs bear the body's weight and give us balance and movement. This means that, unlike the arms, which can maximize their dexterity, the legs have to be strong and very secure. To do this, the legs are made up of thick, strong bones, large muscles that can bear a huge load, joints filled with shock-absorbing cartilage and flat, strong feet and ankles to maximize balance.

Bones

The legs start at the hip, which is a ball and socket joint that fits neatly inside a hole in the pelvic girdle. The femur, the large, long bone at the top of the leg, runs from the hip to the knee, where it becomes wider and meets the tibia, the large bone that runs

down the centre of the lower leg, and the fibula, the smaller bone that allows the lower leg to carry more load as it twists and moves over the ankle. At the ankle, the tibia and fibula meet to join up with the bones of the foot in a joint that relies heavily on ligaments.

BELOW **By keeping the leg muscles flexible and strong, the joints of the knees and ankles are supported.**

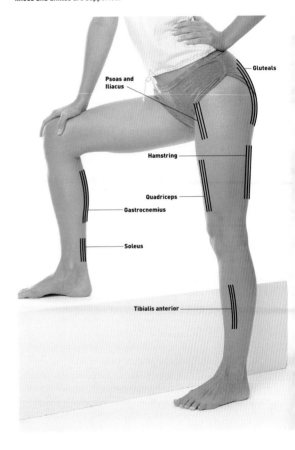

Gluteals

Psoas and Iliacus

Hamstring

Quadriceps

Gastrocnemius

Soleus

Tibialis anterior

Muscles

Just like the arms, the legs contain several major muscle groups, each performing specific functions and working with each other to extend and to facilitate the range of movement.

- The gluteal muscles run from the lower back to the thigh, forming the major muscle groups of the buttocks. When these muscles contract they pull on the femur to straighten the leg from the hip.
- The psoas and iliacus muscles run down the front of the hip from the side of the body; they bend the leg from the hip.
- The hamstring muscles at the back of the thigh contract to bend the knee.
- The quadriceps muscles at the front of the thigh contract to straighten the knee (a sheet of strong tendonous tissue called the iliotibial band runs down the outside of the thigh to help stabilize this movement).
- The muscles at the back of the calf, including the gastrocnemius and the soleus, contract to point the foot.
- The muscles of the shin, including the tibialis anterior, contract to bring the toes towards the shin.

Blood and nerve supply

It is important to understand the location of nerves before beginning massage. The major arteries serving the leg run through the centre of the hip, travelling down the middle of the thigh (femoral artery) and through the back of the knee (popliteal artery) before branching out into the lower leg and foot. The major nerves (sciatic nerve, femoral nerve and peroneal nerves) run down from the bottom of the spine through the hip and branch out to cover the muscles and skin surface.

Lymphatic drainage

The arms and legs hold the major lymphatic drainage systems of the body, which carry lymph and fluid to be dealt with in the lymph glands. This body system serves to reduce swelling and drain fluid from the limbs and is particularly important for people who spend long periods standing upright, as gravity can cause collections of fluid in the lower limbs.

Massage boosts lymphatic drainage in several ways; first, application of pressure and strokes can reduce blockages and free up sticky channels; second, the act of stroking upwards actually 'pushes' fluid up the lymph vessels; and third, the general increase in circulation that follows massage helps fluid transfer in individual cells and tissues. Because of the dramatic effects massage can have on lymphatic drainage, it is important that it is performed correctly. As such it can give your body a massive boost; used incorrectly or in the wrong order it can cause blockage, fluid build-up and pain. Massage should work from the top down, using upward strokes. This means that:

- The individual strokes of the massage should always move in an upward direction, from the extremeties towards the heart, to push lymph and fluid upwards.
- Clearing techniques should start at the top of the limb and work downwards, clearing the lymph from the top to avoid fluid build-up.
- Even though the massager starts at the top, the techniques stroke upwards.

RIGHT **When performing a massage to enhance lymphatic drainage, work from the hands and feet towards the heart, following the arrows as shown here.**

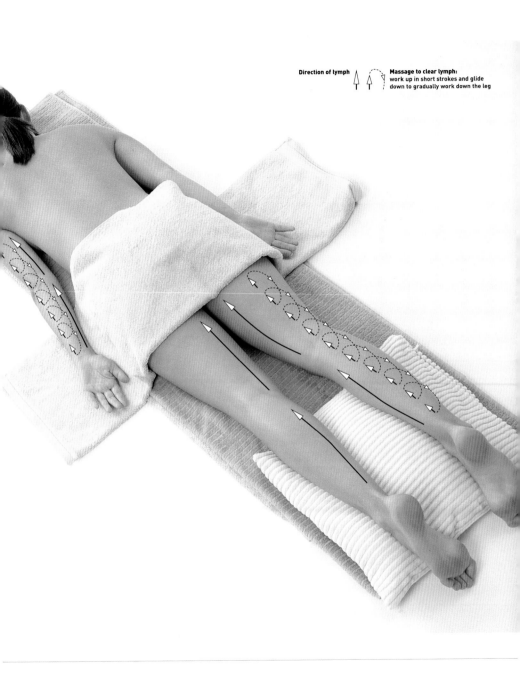

Direction of lymph

Massage to clear lymph:
work up in short strokes and glide
down to gradually work down the leg

BEFORE THE NEXT technique, make sure the body is lying supine – face up.

▼ Front of shoulder effleurage

To ease tension in the postural muscles at the front of the shoulder, especially good for people who work at keyboards.

1. Face the left side of the person's chest.
2. With your left hand, lift up and support the arm so that it lies out at a ninety-degree angle to the body, elbow slightly bent.
3. Place your right thumb on the front of the shoulder where it meets the arm.
4. Make a stroke up from the shoulder towards the collarbone, stopping gently when your thumb reaches the bone.

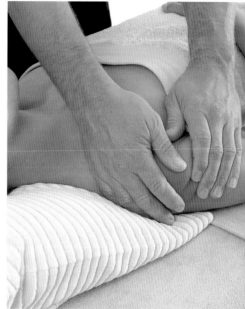

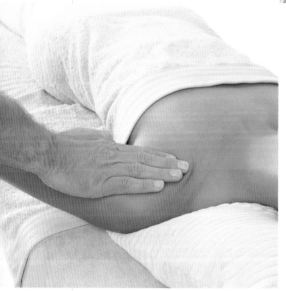

▲ Top of shoulder petrissage

To reduce stress and postural tension on top of the shoulder and into the neck.

1. Face the left shoulder at an angle to the body.
2. Place both hands on top of the shoulder so that the palms cover either side.
3. Petrissage by bringing thumb and forefinger together at the same time as exerting slight pressure downwards, pressing hard enough to produce a redness, and a slight torquing of the skin as your hands move over it.

▼ Bicep effleurage

To stimulate flow of blood and lymph in the upper arm and boost circulation.

1 Face the left arm.
2 With your left hand, pick up and support the forearm so that the elbow is slightly bent, and the inside of the upper arm – the bicep – is exposed.
3 With your right hand, form a slight curve around the upper arm at elbow level (your thumb should be close to the elbow) and then allow your fingers to fall and relax so they conform to the shape of the arm.
4 Make a firm stroke up the arm towards the shoulder, leading with the outside edge of the palm, until you reach the crook of the arm.

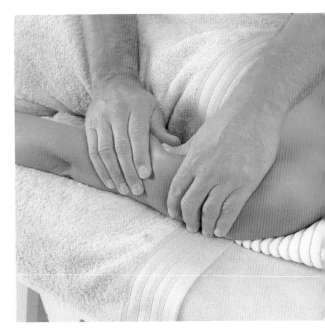

▲ Bicep petrissage

To work deeper into the arm muscles to reduce tension.

1 Place both hands on the top of the arm at the elbow and petrissage in an upward direction, working slowly towards the shoulder.

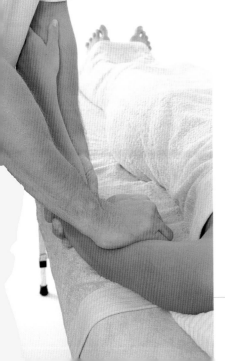

tip It is important to remember that the movement of your hands to petrissage should come from a rolling action in the hips and legs. The arms and shoulders should remain locked in position in a relaxed posture.

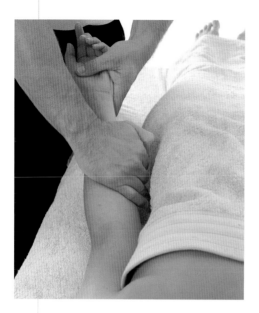

▲ Inside of forearm effleurage

To encourage the flow of lymph and blood away from the hand towards the heart and to boost circulation in the lower arm.

1   Face the bottom of the left arm.
2   With your left hand, raise the arm by the hand so that it is bent, and the wrist and hand lie directly above the elbow in a vertical line with muscles relaxed.
3   With your right hand, form a conformable shape over the top of the forearm at the wrist and make a firm stroke down towards the elbow
4   Repeat the stroke at both sides of the forearm, moving about 5 cm (2 in) in either direction to cover the whole forearm in three strokes.

▼ Palm stretching

To reduce stress and strain in the muscles and soft tissue of the hands and increase flexibility.

1   Face the left hand.
2   With both hands, pick up the hand so that the palm faces up, towards the ceiling, with your fingers at the back of the hand and your two thumbs resting in the middle of the palm touching each other.
3   Slowly draw the thumbs apart, at the same time as flexing the hands slightly back and outwards, so that you stretch the palm out as the thumbs move away from each other.

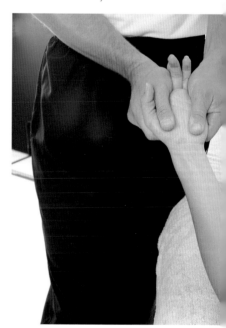

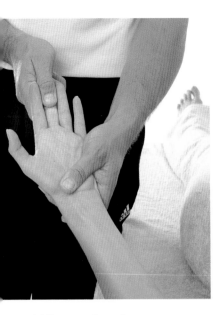

▼ Base of thumb petrissage

To work deep into the large muscles at the base of the thumb.

1 Place your right hand into the hand so that the creases between thumbs and first fingers lie touching each other. Adjust your position by moving your hand up and down until your thumb sits flat on the fleshy part at the base of the thumb and your fingers support the area behind the base of the thumb.

2 Move your thumb in small circular clockwise movements around the base of the thumb so that it works into the muscle.

▲ Finger drawing

To ease away tension held in the hands.

1 With your left hand, support the forearm so that the elbow is bent and the arm muscles are relaxed.

2 Place the right hand over the first finger of the hand so the thumb points down the hand and the fingers curl loosely around the back of the finger.

3 Draw the finger out by exerting a slight pull as you draw your hand down the finger, with the thumb working down the inside of the finger and the fingers down the outside.

4 At the same time as you draw the finger out, move the hand up and down in a rocking motion to maximize the relaxation and stretch benefits.

5 Work your way down the fingers, repeating the process for each finger.

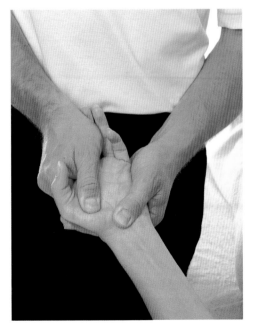

▼ Back of forearm effleurage

To stimulate the flow of blood and lymph up the forearm and clear fluid blockages.

1 Face the left hand of the person being massaged.
2 With your own left hand, pick up the arm by the hand so that it is bent and the wrist and hand lie vertically above the elbow with muscles relaxed.

3 With your right hand form a conformable shape over the top of the forearm at the wrist and along one side of the forearm – the cupped shape of the hand should follow the contours of the forearm.
4 Make a firm, slow stroke towards the elbow. Do not allow the wrist to bend.
5 Repeat the stroke at both sides of the forearm, moving about 5 cm (2 in) in either direction to cover the whole forearm in three strokes.

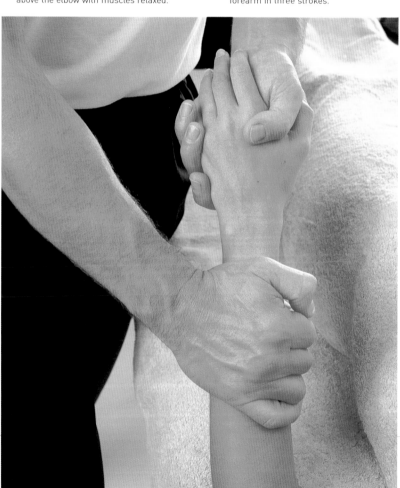

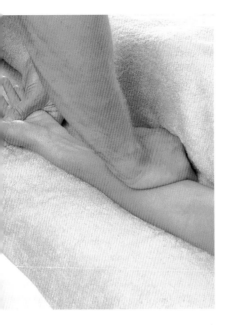

▲ Anterior forearm compression

To work into the muscles of the forearm to help reduce muscle tension and release toxins.

1   Using the heel of your hand, press down for a few seconds at the wrist end of the forearm, then release the pressure and move up 3–5 cm (1–2 in).
2   Continue this, pressing, releasing and moving up until you have covered the whole back surface of the forearm and reached the elbow.

▼ Forearm STR

To stretch specific parts of the muscles of the forearm.

1   Position yourself by the left forearm.
2   With your left hand, extend the hand to contract the muscle on top of the forearm. It should be extended but not stretched and should feel comfortable.
3   With your right hand, push the thumb directly into the muscle on top of the arm with a downward movement.
4   Move the thumb upwards (towards the elbow) by about 1.5 cm (½ in), so that you stretch the muscle slightly underneath it.
5   Lock the thumb in position and, slowly and gently, move the hand back down.

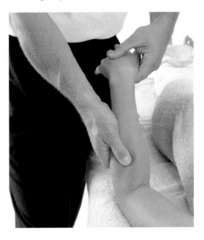

tip The point of contact where the thumb meets the muscle might be a little sore because this is a deep technique that stretches the muscle. It should not be painful except for a mild feeling of discomfort or tenderness where the thumb is in contact. If it causes pain or soreness, stop immediately and move on to another massage.

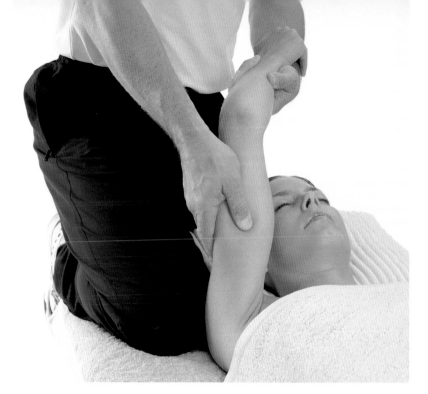

Bicep petrissage

**To work deep into the muscles of the
top of the arm to boost circulation and
release tension.**

1   Face the left elbow.
2   Place both hands on the top of the
    arm at the bicep, with palms of hands
    on top of the arm and the fingers
    pointing downwards.
3   Grasping the skin and exerting a
    gentle downward pressure, bring
    alternate thumbs and fingers together
    to petrissage the bicep muscle.
4   Move the petrissage around so you
    cover the whole area between the
    elbow and the shoulder.

▲ Tricep STR

**To target specific parts of the muscle
for localized stretching.**

1   With the left hand, hold the forearm
    straight up in the air without lifting the
    shoulder – straighten, do not stretch.
2   Push the thumb of your right hand,
    directly into the muscle at the back
    of the arm (the tricep) near the back of
    the elbow. Lock the thumb in place
    and, keeping the same pressure, move
    it down towards the shoulder so that
    the muscle is locally stretched.
3   Keeping the thumb in place, stretch
    further by using your left arm to bend
    the arm at the elbow, releasing your
    thumb as the hand gets to the shoulder.
4   Repeat several times as you work your
    way towards the armpit.

BEFORE THE NEXT technique, direct the person being massaged to turn face down.

▼ Tricep effleurage I

To encourage the flow of lymph, blood and toxins away from the back of the arm.

1   Face the right side of the person being massaged.
2   Using your left hand, grasp the forearm and bend the elbow inwards.
3   Place your right hand over the tricep at the back of the arm, with the palm of the hand facing downwards and the side of the hand at the elbow forming a contour over the arm.
4   Stroke your hand towards the shoulder, using the palm to produce pressure on the tricep.

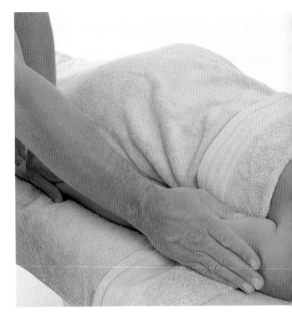

▲ Tricep effleurage II

To work away tension and toxins from the upper arm.

1   Face the right ribcage with your body at forty-five degrees to the arm.
2   Bring the arm down so that it lies palm up by their side.
3   Place the thumb of your right hand on the tricep at the elbow and make a long stroke down towards the shoulder. Use the thumb to exert pressure and allow the fingers to form a contour around the arm shape.
4   Move your hand slightly to left and right and repeat the stroke.

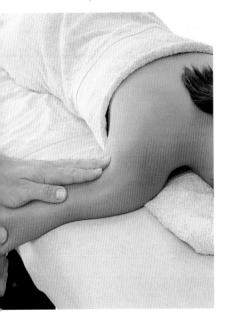

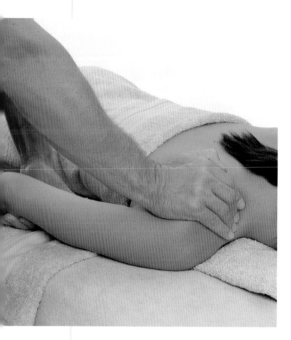

BEFORE THE NEXT technique, direct the person being massaged to turn onto their back so that the massage can be performed with the body lying supine – face up.

▶ Complete arm shake for relaxation

To relax the muscles at the end of the massage and to encourage all the tissues and fibres of the arm to work together to reduce toxins and tension and to boost relaxation, regeneration and healing. The arm shake should be used following all arm massages.

1   Stand slightly apart from the body at hip level, facing at an angle to the body so that you look directly towards the shoulder.
2   Using both hands, grasp the sides of the wrist and hand and lift the arm about 10 cm (4 in) so that the elbow and upper arm are supported and the shoulder is not lifted off the ground.
3   Using both arms together, make gentle up and down movements to shake the whole arm in a relaxed and controlled motion, starting with larger movements that get smaller and smaller until they stop.

▲ Back of shoulder effleurage

To ease tension in the postural muscles and stimulate circulation.

1   Lie the arm, palm up, by their side. Place your left hand in the crook of the elbow and lift about 5 cm (2 in) to reveal the shoulder blade.
2   Place the palm of your right hand flat on the top of the arm by the shoulder with your fingers pointing towards the shoulder. Lift the fingers slightly and stroke with the palm towards the top of the shoulder and into the shoulder blade, stopping level with the armpit.
3   Repeat several times, pushing harder each time.

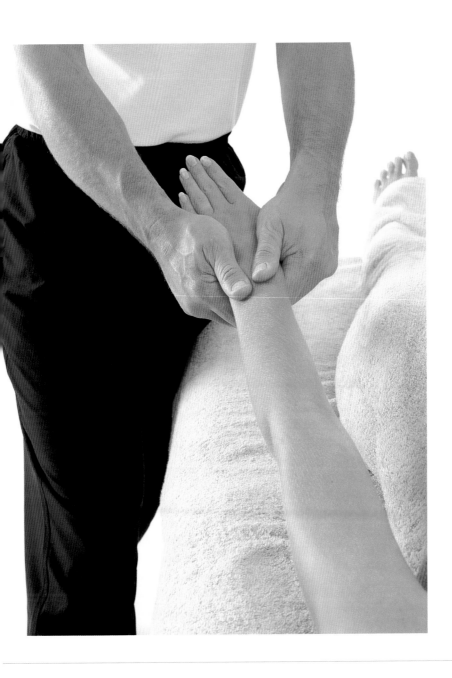

Complete arm shake

▼ Rolling compressions working down the thigh

To prepare the muscles in the front of the thigh for deep massage by clearing lymph, fluid and toxin build-up.

1 Position yourself halfway up the left thigh facing up towards the head.
2 Place both hands, palm down on the top of the thigh with fingers slightly raised and the right hand a fraction higher up the thigh than the left.
3 Press with the heel of your right hand, hold for a few seconds and release.
4 Repeat with the left hand, then move the right hand down and repeat, pressing and releasing with alternate hands all the way down the thigh to release tension.

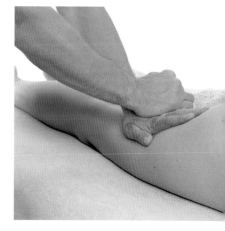

▲ Heel of hand thigh compressions

To clear more toxins, lymph and tension.

1 Place your left hand palm down, fingers raised, in the centre of the thigh, 5 cm (2 in) below the groin.
2 Place the right hand on top of the left so that the heel of the right hand is directly above the heel of the left.
3 Lock your wrists so they do not move.
4 Make a deep stroke of about 7.5 cm (3 in) using the heel of your hands to apply pressure in an upward direction.
5 Move down 15 cm (6 in) and make another stroke, the same length as the first and ending where the first began.
6 Continue to work down the thigh, making deep strokes of about 7.5 cm (3 in) in length all the way down. The strokes should not overlap and should end where the previous one began.
7 Once you reach the soft muscle on top of the knee, move your hands to the top inside of the thigh and repeat. Do the same for the outside of the thigh.

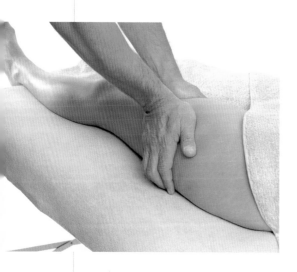

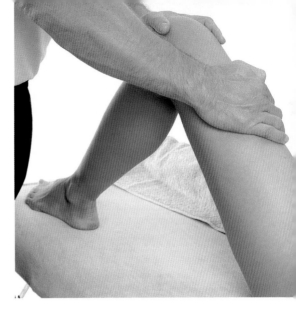

▼ Thigh effleurage I

To encourage the flow of lymph away from the leg and boost circulation.

1 Position yourself beside the left knee facing towards the head.
2 Place your left hand over the fleshy muscle on top of the knee so the side of your hand faces up towards the head and your thumb lies alongside the fingers nearest to the knee.
3 Assume the lunge position and place your right hand over the top of your left hand, slightly further back towards the knee so the last two fingers of the left hand are not covered.
4 Lunge forwards and make a single stroke up from the knee to the top of the thigh, pushing down with the side of your hand and allowing your hand to follow the contours of the thigh to maximize the point of contact. Finish the stroke at the top of the thigh.

▲ Thigh effleurage II

To release deep tension contained in the thigh muscles.

1 Bend the knee and put the foot flat on the bed or floor surface to stretch the thigh muscle.
2 Steady the leg with your left hand.
3 With your right hand lying across the thigh, make a single stroke up from the knee to the top of the thigh, pushing down with the side of your hand and allowing your hand to follow the contours of the thigh to maximize the point of contact.
4 Finish the stroke at the top of the thigh in a controlled manner.
5 Replace the leg to its lying position, with the knee straight or slightly bent.

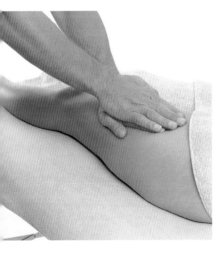

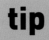**tip** While performing this technique, do not touch the kneecap itself. Start above the knee and work gently upwards.

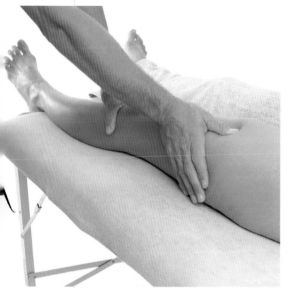

▼ Thigh petrissage

To work over the whole thigh to boost circulation to all muscles and soft tissues, as well as to encourage the regeneration of the skin and the release of tension.

1   Face the right thigh.
2   Reach over and place both hands next to each other palm down on the left thigh just above, but not touching, the knee with fingers and thumbs forming a loose triangle.
3   Bring alternate fingers to thumbs to petrissage and move up the thigh, working from the knee to the hip up the outside of the thigh.

▲ Deep effleurage of thigh

To work deep into the thigh muscles targeting specific areas for circulation and regeneration.

1   Place your right hand on the thigh, just above the knee, so that the fingers point down the outside of the thigh towards the head and the thumb rests on top of the thigh.
2   Make a deep stroke upwards in a straight line, continuing up the centre of the thigh from the knee to the hip. Use your fingers to guide the stroke.
3   Repeat the stroke from above the knee a further four times, twice on the inside of the thigh and then twice on the outside. Do not go over the same part of the thigh twice.

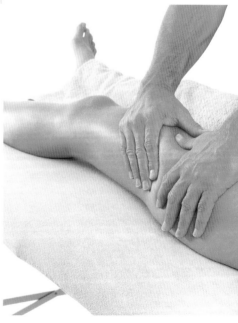

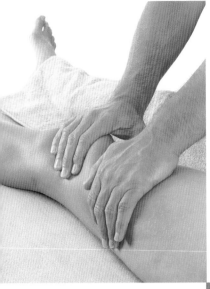

▼ Ankle to knee effleurage

To boost the flow of lymph, to increase circulation and to ease away tension.

1   Position yourself about halfway down the left shin.
2   Place your left hand over the very bottom of the shin, just above but not on the ankle, with the side of the hand facing up towards the head and the thumb on the side nearest the foot.
3   With the heel of your right hand, lunge forward to make a single stroke from ankle to knee. Finish underneath the knee without touching the kneecap.
4   Repeat several times, moving to the outside and inside of the shin.

▲ Transverse draw of knee ligaments

To work across the knee ligament, which can become tight, and to free up tension in the centre of the leg.

1   Reach over with your left hand and form a loose hook with fingers, at the bottom of the thigh above the knee.
2   Place your right palm on top of the left hand, lock wrists, arms and shoulders.
3   Pull with the left hand while applying pressure down through the palm with the right to stretch the knee ligaments under your fingers, work in an arc to finish on top of the thigh about 5 cm (2 in) higher than where you started.
4   Move about 5 cm (2 in) up the leg and repeat the draw parallel to the first one, continuing to move up and repeat until you reach the top of the thigh.

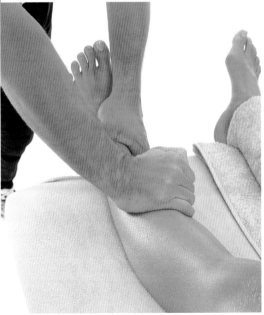

▼ Shin STR

To target specific areas of the shin muscle, easing away stresses and strains and boosting flexibility.

1. Using the left hand, flex the foot so that the toes point to the ceiling and your palm supports the foot sole.
2. With your right thumb, press into the centre of the muscle that runs down the front of the shin, just to the side of the bone, and lock the thumb in position. Then move upwards towards the knee while still exerting pressure.
3. Use the left hand to bring the foot slowly to a point, while keeping the right thumb in position to increase the stretch.
4. Repeat several times over the muscle; do not press into the same area twice.

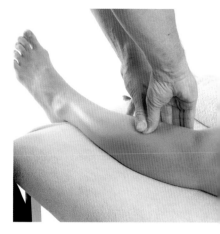

▲ Transverse glide across front of shin

To work deeper into the muscles at the front of the shin, which are prone to tension, to ease away fibrous build up and separate it from surrounding tissues to clear away toxins.

1. Place your thumbs pointing towards you beside the shin bone on the muscle that runs up beside the shin, just below the knee. Your fingers should be pointing down the inside of the lower leg.
2. Dropping your bodyweight, make a single stroke down towards you, pulling the shin directly away from the shinbone. Stop the stroke when you feel your thumbs coming off the edge of the shin.
3. Move down about 5 cm (2 in) and repeat the stroke, working towards the ankle, until you have covered the whole shin.

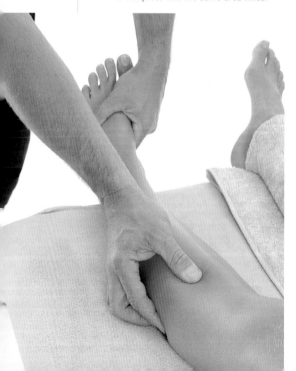

▼ Draw of front of foot

To work into the muscles, ligaments and tendons of the foot in order to stretch and ease tension.

1 Position yourself by the left foot facing the head.
2 Grasp the ankle with your right hand so that the thumbs sit on top of the foot and the fingers and palm support the sole. Hold the shin steady with your left hand.
3 Lock your wrists, arms and shoulders in position and rock back on your feet, pushing apart with your thumbs at the same time so your right hand stretches the foot sideways while your left stretches it lengthways.
4 Repeat several times to stretch out the ligaments and tendons of the foot.

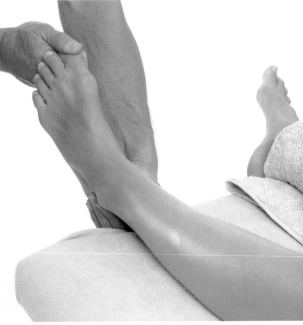

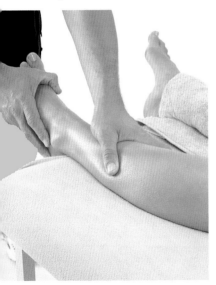

▲ Toe stretch

To work into the toes for nervous stimulation to boost balance and skin regeneration.

1 With the left hand, support the left foot at the heel, lifting it about 5 cm (2 in).
2 Place the right thumb on top of the base of the little toe and curl your right index finger underneath the toe at the base.
3 Slowly and gently draw the toe out, using the finger as a pivot and the thumb to stretch the toe out over the top of it.
4 Repeat for each toe.

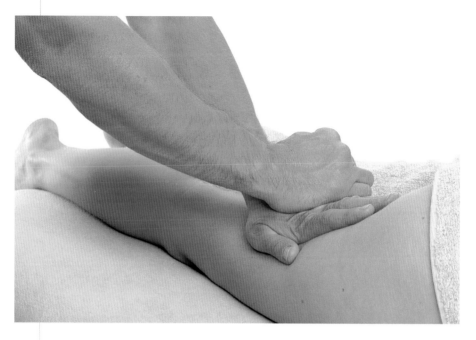

BEFORE YOU BEGIN the following techniques, direct the person being massaged to turn onto their stomach so that the body is lying prone (facing the floor).

▲ Heel of hand working down hamstrings

1 Position yourself beside the left thigh facing the head.
2 Place your left palm on the centre of the thigh, 5 cm (2 in) below the bottom, with fingers slightly raised.
3 Place the right hand on top of the left so that the heel of the right hand is directly above the heel of the left.
4 Lock your wrists together. Make a deep stroke of about 7.5 cm (3 in) using the heel of your hands to apply pressure in an upward direction.

5 Move the hands down 15 cm (6 in) and make another stroke (this stroke should be the same length as the first and should end where the first began).
6 Continue to work down the thigh in this way, pushing upwards but working downwards to clear the lymph, making deep strokes of about 7.5 cm (3 in) in length all the way.
7 Stop compressions BEFORE you reach the soft triangle behind and above the knee (the location of the leg artery, which should never be massaged).
8 Move your hands to the top inside of the thigh and repeat. Repeat again for the outside of the thigh.

tip After the first stroke with your hands, you can do this with your forearm. Get close to the body with your shoulder over the leg. Bend your elbow directly under your shoulder, hold the left wrist with the right hand and stroke up using the forearm.

▼ Hamstrings effleurage I

1 Position yourself by the left knee facing the head of the person being massaged.
2 Place your left hand palm down on the bottom of the hamstrings (avoiding the soft fleshy triangle at the back of the knee where the main leg artery is located). Place it sideways so that the thumb is nearest the knee, and cover it with your right hand.
3 If you are at a massage table or bed, move one of your legs forward to give you a stable base to lunge onto, and lunge forward, making a stroke up the thigh towards the head.

▼ Cam and spindle of the hamstrings

1 Form a fist with your left hand. Place it knuckle down on the the back of the thigh, 7.5 cm (3 in) below the buttocks.
2 Place the thumb of the right hand inside the left fist and the palm of the right hand flat on the outside of the thigh with fingers pointing to the head.
3 Use the right hand as a guide and the left fist for pressure, make a short stroke up towards the head.
4 At the end of the stroke move about 15 cm (6 in) down the thigh and repeat, continue down the thigh. Stop before you reach the soft triangle at the back of the knee.

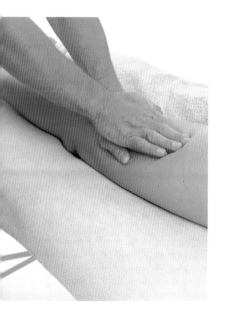

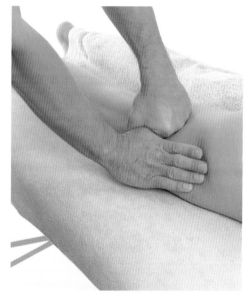

▼ Hamstrings effleurage II

1 Place your left thumb on the bottom of the hamstrings (avoid the soft fleshy triangle at the back of the knee) and cover it with the right thumb.
2 Move one of your legs forward to give you a stable base to lunge onto and lunge forward, making a deep thumb stroke up the thigh towards the head.
3 Repeat several times to the left and right of the original stroke, taking care not to cover the same area twice.

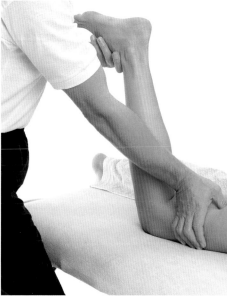

▲ Hamstrings STR

1 Position yourself by the left hamstrings facing the feet.
2 With your left hand, pick up the foot so that the knee bends and the foot points straight up towards the ceiling.
3 Put the right thumb into the hamstring muscle about halfway up the leg and shift it backwards up to the head about 5 cm (2 in) to put the muscle on a stretch.
4 Using your left hand for control, slowly drop the foot so the knee straightens and the hamstring is stretched.
5 Repeat several times, working the whole thigh but carefully avoiding the fleshy soft triangle above the back of the knee.

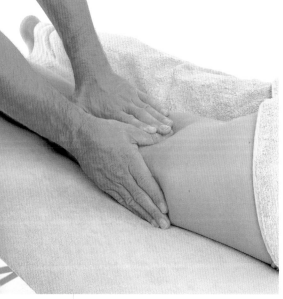

▼ Rolling compressions of the calf

1 Position yourself by the left calf facing the head.
2 Place both hands palm down on top of the calf below the knee with the fingers slightly raised and the right hand slightly higher up than the left.
3 Press down with the heel of your right hand, hold for a few seconds and then gently release.
4 Repeat with the left hand and then move the right hand down and repeat, pressing and releasing with alternate hands, working the whole way down the calf to the ankle.

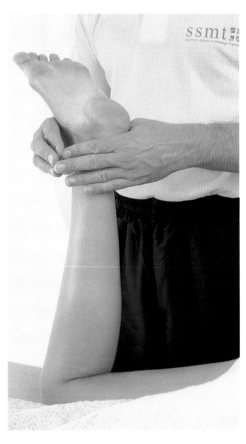

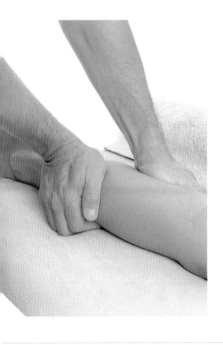

▲ Side calf vibrations

1 Position yourself by the left knee and pick up the foot, bending the knee so that the foot points to the ceiling.
2 Use both hands to form a loose circle with fingers and thumbs around the ankle and let the foot rock in this circle to gently vibrate the calf muscle.

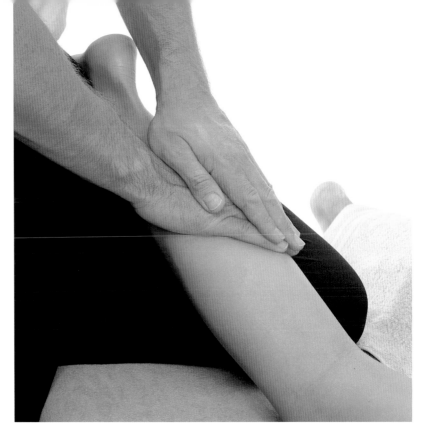

▲ Calf effleurage I

1 Position yourself by the right calf facing the head. Arrange the leg so the knee is bent and the calf is resting on your knee, a towel or a cushion – the foot should be higher than the knee and hip.
2 Put your right hand over the calf at the ankle, with the outside of the hand facing towards the knee, and cover it with the left hand.
3 Firmly stroke up the calf from ankle to knee, finishing in the crook of the knee.

Calf effleurage II

1 Place your left thumb just above the ankle with the outside of the hand facing up towards the knee. Cover the thumb with the right hand so that the last two fingers of the left hand are not covered.
2 Make a firm stroke up the calf from ankle to knee, finishing in the crook of the knee.

▶ Sole of foot effleurage

1 Position yourself by the right foot.
2 Put both thumbs on the sole of
   the foot by the toes, and support the
   underside with the palms and fingers.
3 Make a deep stroke with your thumbs
   down from the toes towards the heel.

▼ Knuckle kneading to
sole of foot

1 Support the front of the foot with
   the left hand, and then place the
   right hand in a loose fist on the sole
   of the foot.
2 Using the knuckles, knead into the
   sole, working up from heel to toes.

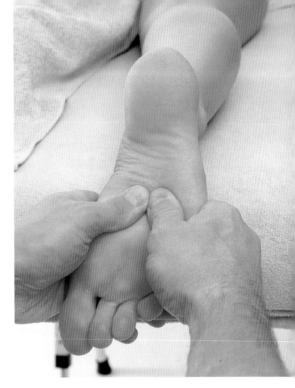

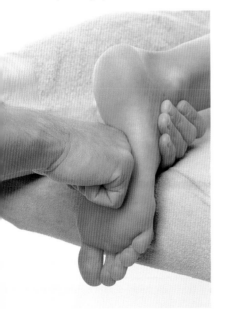

Complete leg relaxation
vibrations

1 Hold the foot with one hand under the
   heel and one hand on top of the foot.
2 Tighten your grip slightly and arrange
   your hands so that they hold the foot
   secure at the ankle and no twisting is
   possible.
3 Shake your hands gently up and
   down to produce a vibration up the
   whole leg.
4 Repeat with a side-to-side motion of
   your hands for total relaxation.

Complete leg relaxation vibrations

Abdominal
and Rib Massage

The midpoint of our body holds the key

to many of our vital life processes. It is often

this area that responds to stressful situations in

our lives and holding the trunk in tension can cause

problems with digestion and other vital processes. Not only does the

abdomen contain the digestive system which absorbs nutrients and

energy from the food and water we consume, but it also holds

the kidneys, liver, spleen and, in women, the reproductive organs.

Massage boosts circulation and removes blockages and toxins

from abdominal soft tissue, as well as helps the gut to work

efficiently by giving the movement of its contents a helping hand.

This chapter shows you how to massage the abdomen to ease

problems with digestion, dissolve away muscle tension and get

rid of breathing problems and rib stiffness. Working through the

techniques from beginning to end will take around 15 minutes.

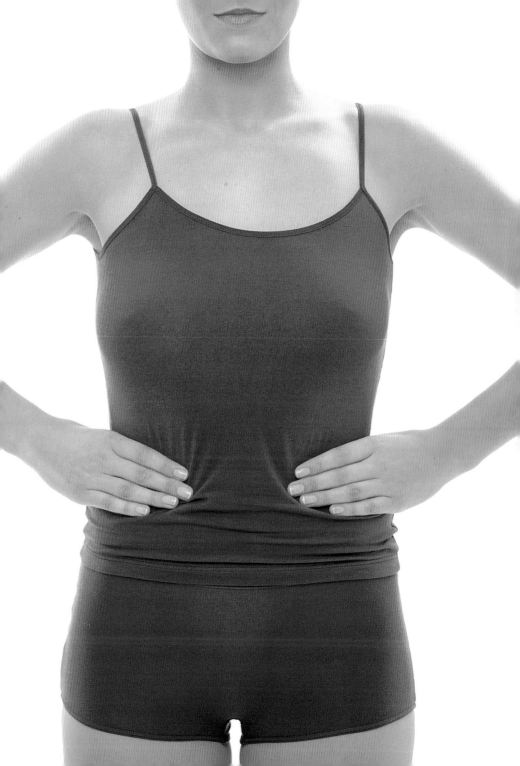

Basic anatomy

The abdominal cavity is home to much more than just the stomach. The liver, kidneys, reproductive organs and the lower half of the digestive tract are all securely contained here, so massage can be very beneficial for general health and wellbeing.

The digestive system

Food is broken down into an easily digestible form in the stomach, and then travels into the small intestine, where nutrients and

BELOW **Be aware of the position of the internal organs, diaphragm and colon in the abdomen when massaging.**

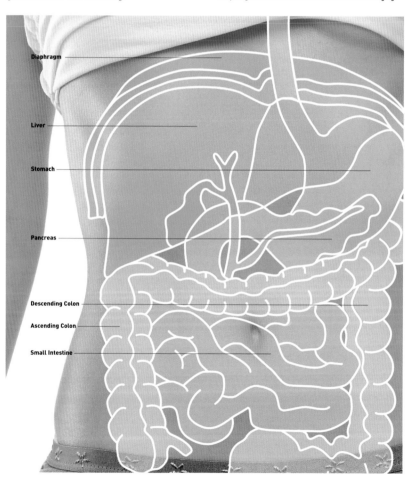

Diaphragm

Liver

Stomach

Pancreas

Descending Colon

Ascending Colon

Small Intestine

energy are absorbed. The small intestine is composed of a tube that runs from the ribs to the lower abdomen in twisting rows. The food travels down this until it reaches the end, near the right hip. It then enters the large intestine, which is where the last stages of digestion and most of the water absorption take place. The large intestine has three main parts – an ascending arm which runs up the right side of the body from the front of the hip to the bottom of the ribcage, a small part which runs across the bottom of the ribcage and a descending arm which runs from the ribcage down the left side, finishing above the left hip and emptying into the rectum.

Food travels through all parts of the intestine by a motion called peristalsis, which is a contraction of the circular muscle of the

NOTE

It is very important when massaging that the strokes never oppose the movement of food through the gut, as this could cause blockage, toxin build-up and digestive problems. Clearance strokes should move from the right hip up towards the ribs, across and down the left side, following the direction of the large colon. Abdominal massage should never use too much force as it could damage important organs underneath the skin – it should be firm but soft and should certainly never cause any pain or discomfort.

vessel walls. In some sections, such as the ascending arm of the large colon, this muscle activity is working against gravity. Massage in these areas can help to increase the efficiency of the digestive processes.

The ribs and diaphragm

The ribs, and the intercostal muscles that allow them to move against each other, are vital for efficient functioning of the body. When we breathe in, the diaphragm – a strong but thin sheet of fibrous material that sits under the ribcage – is forced down into the abdominal cavity and the ribcage expands, forcing oxygenated air into the lungs. When we breathe out, the ribs collapse back, the diaphragm is sucked into the chest and the air in the lungs is expelled. Breathing problems can be debilitating and upsetting, but massage of the intercostal muscles and the bottom of the ribcage helps to release any build up of tension and toxins that can affect breathing. The soothing strokes also deepen breathing and encourage relaxation.

Finding the right position

Positioning for abdominal massage is different to that for other types because it is important that the abdominal muscles are relaxed and not put on a stretch. Sometimes when we lie flat on our backs the abdomen can be stretched, decreasing not only comfort but also the efficiency of the massage. To make sure the abdomen is perfectly relaxed, the person being massaged should lie on their back facing the ceiling, with a pillow under their head to raise it up slightly (but keeping the neck straight). Another pillow should be placed under the knees so the legs are bent slightly at the hip and the curve of the lower back is just in contact with the floor. This should free up the abdominal muscles from doing any work, allowing them to relax.

Unlike the techniques for the back, neck, shoulders, arms and legs, these abdominal massages cover the whole area, so there is no need to repeat them on the other side.

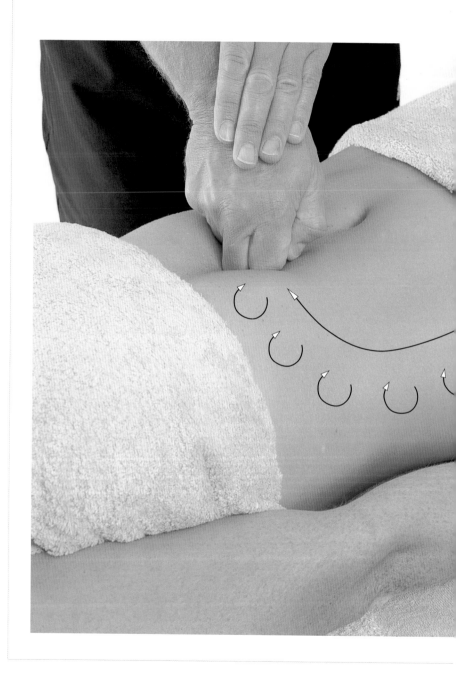

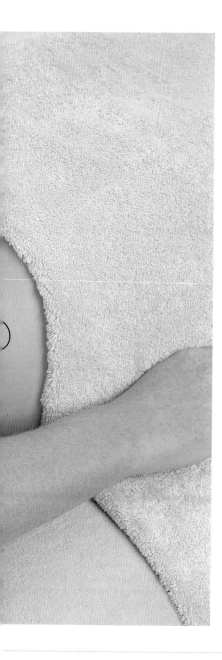

BEFORE THE FOLLOWING techniques, make sure the person being massaged is lying supine – face up.

◀Clockwise circular stroking

1. Position yourself by the abdomen, facing the head of the person being massaged.
2. Place your right hand lightly on the abdomen just above the right hip and form a very loose fist so that the knuckles are in contact with the skin.
3. Taking care not to press too hard, work your fist in a small clockwise circle at the right hip, ending the stroke slightly above the position you started in.
4. Move up towards the head about 5 cm (2 in) and repeat the circular stroke (remember to go clockwise).
5. Work your way slowly and gently up the right side of the abdomen to the bottom of the ribcage, across the lower ribcage and down the left side of the abdomen towards the left hip, finishing just above the left hip, level with your starting position.

tip This helps to clear the digestive tract so it is important that all strokes work clockwise and from the right hip up and around to the left, following the direction of the intestine. This stroke must be done before any other abdominal massage.

▼ Alternate hands effleurage

1 Face the left side of the abdomen of the person being massaged.
2 Place both hands palm-down on the abdomen above the right hip with the fingers touching the skin.
3 Using the fingers of the left hand to create light pressure, make an n-shaped stroke in an anticlockwise direction travelling up towards the ribcage on the right side.
4 Make another stroke further up the right side and work your way around the bottom of the ribcage and down towards the left hip, keeping the finger strokes light.

▼ Deep stroking around the bottom of ribs

1 Place your right hand palm-down at the top of the abdomen under the ribcage, so that you can feel the bones at the bottom of the ribcage with the side of your fingers. Cover your right hand with your left hand.
2 Working alongside and just under the bottom of the right side of the ribcage, make deep strokes towards the left side of the body, using the bottom of the ribcage as a guide.

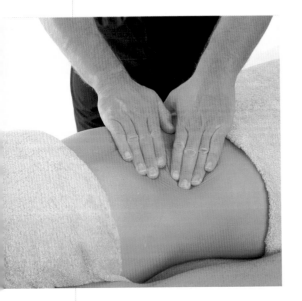

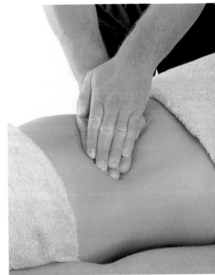

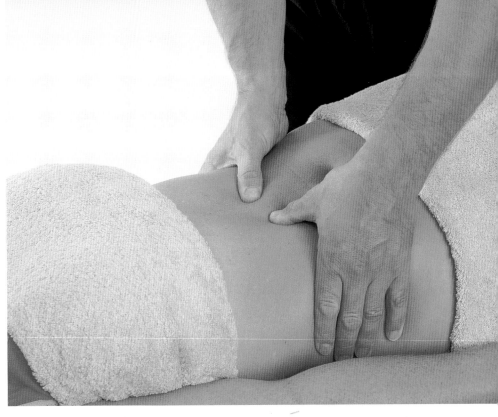

▲ Interactive abdominal compression

1. Position yourself at the left hip, facing the head of the person being massaged.
2. Place your left hand around the side of the body above the hip with the fingers pointing down the side of the body and the thumb positioned so that it sits on top of the abdominal muscles (about 5–7.5 cm (2–3 in) in from the side of the body). Place the right hand in the same position on the opposite side.
3. Ask the person being massaged to bring their head up, using the abdominal muscles, so that they are looking directly down between their feet without twisting or strain.
4. Press your thumbs into the abdominal muscles, then push them upwards and lock in position.
5. Ask the person being massaged to slowly drop their head backwards in a controlled way until the muscles are completely relaxed.
6. Release the thumbs, move a little further up the abdomen and repeat as many times as required until you reach the bottom of the ribcage. Take care not to cover the same area twice.

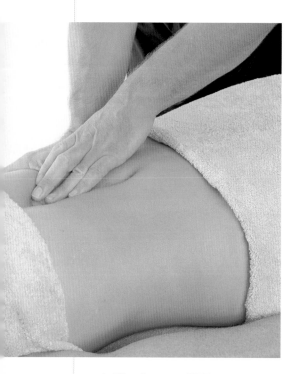

▼ Deep finger rib effleurage

1 Place the right hand on the right side of the ribs, allowing the fingers to fall between the lower ribs at the side.
2 Place your left hand on top of the right fingers and make a stroke, with the fingers staying between the ribs, up towards the centre of the chest.
3 When you reach the centre of the chest, turn the hand over and continue the stroke with the fingers leading the palm down towards the left side (towards your body).

▲ Diaphragm STR

1 Place the right thumb about 10 cm (4 in) away from the centre of the chest just under the bone of the lower rib. Support the thumb using the fingers of your left hand.
2 Ask the person to take a deep breath in, and then as they breathe out push firmly, but not too hard, with your thumb up and under the ribs. Ease off as the out-breath finishes.
3 Repeat twice more, asking them to take longer to breathe out each time.
4 Repeat on the other side.

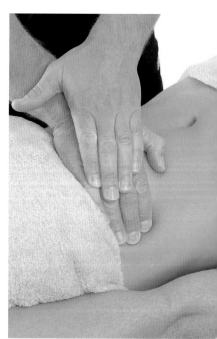

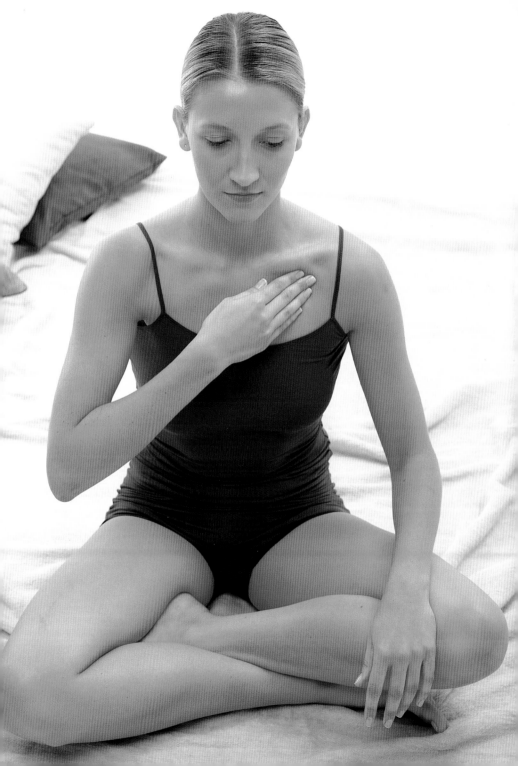

Preparation and tools

Massage soothes, calms and relaxes stressed, tense and tired bodies and boosts overworked minds, but all too often it is not available when we need it most – sitting at a desk, after a gym workout or at home. The great advantage of learning to heal yourself with self-massage is that you can use it any time, anywhere. You don't need to wait for an appointment; just clear your schedule for half an hour and you can reap the beneficial effects of massage when you feel the need.

Tools

There are a variety of self-massage tools that can help you reach hard-to-get-at areas of your body for total tension release.

Chinese balls – Available from oriental shops and some complementary medicine centres, Chinese hand balls are a fun way to keep your hands and fingers flexible. To use them, hold two balls in the palm of a hand

BELOW **Chinese balls can be rolled in the palm of the hand to relieve stress and encourage suppleness.**

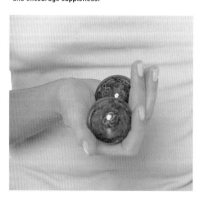

- Stay relaxed, centred and calm. The beneficial effects of the massage will be diminished and even lost if you enter into this personal time in a stressed, frenetic manner.
- Before you start, take at least three long, slow, deep breaths, closing your eyes and concentrating on how the self-treatment massage will benefit your mental and physical states.
- Don't massage or exert pressure if you feel pain in any area.
- Remember to avoid danger zones, such as the soft areas of the eyes, the sides of the neck and the soft triangle above the knee at the back.
- If you are pregnant, or think you might be pregnant, be aware of the possible effects of massage and steer clear of massaging the stomach and lower back. Also avoid the use of essential oils or mediums that may contain them.
- Make that sure your clothing is loose and comfortable and that you occupy a position that allows your back to assume the neutral position, with the neck and head comfortable, supported and not twisted or cricked (see also page 26).
- If you are closing your eyes during the massage, make sure you can't be disturbed – even if it means locking the door or disconnecting your phone.
- Most importantly, never feel guilty about taking a few minutes out to boost your physical and mental state – it is always time worth spending. Learning to give your body and mind what they need allows you to be focused, centred and efficient when you return to daily life.

and circle them around each other using your palm and fingers. Some versions have a musical chime to help relax the mind.

Rubber stress balls – These malleable balls can be squeezed and moulded in your hands to work the muscles and relieve tension.

Massage pegs – Massage pegs fit around the knuckles of the hand and have a roller or ball attached to them for massaging specific points of the body. They can be used for providing light or deep strokes to muscled areas like the thigh, forearm and calf, but care should be taken in bony areas and around joints.

Spiky balls – Soft, spiky rubber balls can help you release tension in your back, neck and shoulders by providing a soft, textured

tip For each of the self-massage techniques, you should start in a relaxed, comfortable position that allows your body to enjoy the massage and your mind to concentrate on the task.

pressure to the muscles. They are most effective if you lie on the floor and place them under your back, neck or shoulders, rolling yourself on top of them in a slow, controlled way to target problem areas and release muscle tension. They can also be rolled under the feet and between the hands.

Foot rollers – Foot rollers are designed to target tension and muscle tiredness in the soles of the feet. Sit in a chair with your foot flat and roll it forwards and backwards over the roller to relieve pain and stiffness.

BELOW **Rollers for the hands and feet can be used to target stiff and sore areas.**

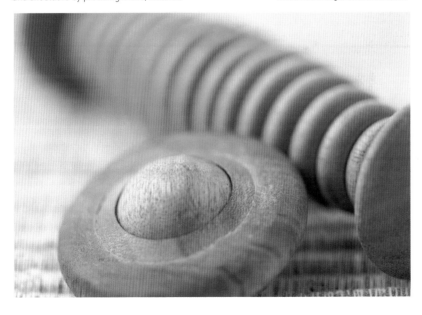

THE FOLLOWING TECHNIQUES help to relieve the pain and pressure of headaches, migraines and sinus problems.

▼ Temple massage

To relax the eyes, forehead and scalp, reducing stress and soothing away the pain of tension headaches.

1   Place the flats of your thumbs on the temples. They should sit comfortably in the dip between the outside of the eyebrow and the hairline.
2   Exert gentle pressure on the temples and move the hands simultaneously towards the eyebrow in a circular motion, working from the hairline towards the eye, past the eyebrow and back up towards the hairline. Make sure you cover the whole space of the temple with your fingers.
3   Continue this circular movement for at least a minute, closing your eyes and concentrating on releasing tension in the forehead and eyes.

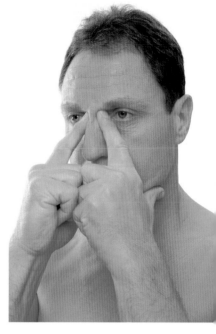

▲ Circular sinus compressions

Soothes and revitalizes tired and stressed eyes to reduce headache pain and release tension.

1   Place the first fingers of each hand either side of the top of the bridge of the nose, the area where it curves up into the eyebrow.
2   Using gentle pressure, make circular motions on both sides, closing the eyes as you do this.
3   Repeat these circular motions for at least a minute.

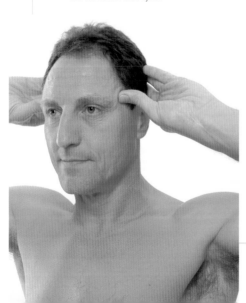

▼ Occiput thumb compressions

1   Place the flats of the thumbs behind the bottom of the ears under the skull bone (which will feel round under your thumb) and reach your fingers to the crown of your head.

2   Trace the line of the bottom of the skull around towards the spine until you reach a soft area under the skull (about 5 cm (2 in) around from the spine). This area is called the occiput.

3   Gently press the thumbs into the occiput and make small circular motions, working upwards closer into the spine and then downwards nearer the ear.

4   Continue these circular occiput compressions for at least a minute.

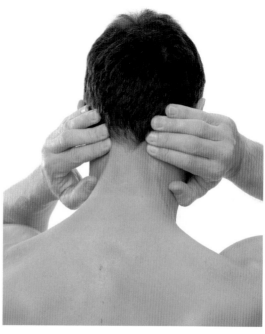

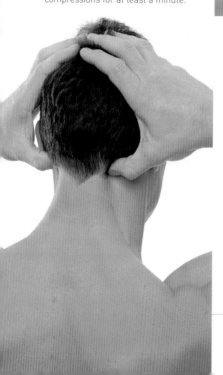

▲ Occiput draw

1   Position both palms to touch the skin on the side of the neck, cupping the ears and with the fingers reaching up towards the occiput.

2   Exert pressure on the occiput with the first two fingers, drawing them across the edge of the spine towards the ear. Palms should rest on the sides of the neck.

3   Bring your chin down and in so the neck is stretched throughout the draw.

4   Stop the draw when your fingers reach the area behind the ears and repeat the whole movement several times.

tip A major cause of headaches is tension and stress stored at the top of the neck, where it meets the skull at the back of the head, the occiput. This massage releases tension to soothe away pain and stress in this area.

Ice massage

This technique is designed to reduce inflammation and pain through the application and soothing massage of ice. Always wrap ice up in a soft material or it could cause cold burns to the skin.

1   Prepare an ice pack by wrapping up several ice cubes in a linen towel or an absorbent cloth. Alternatively buy a ready-made pack.
2   Rub the ice pack gently on the back of your neck, the base of your skull and the forehead and temples, using slow circular movements to soothe away inflammation.
3   Never continue the massage for longer than five minutes – the maximum time for ice massage in this area.

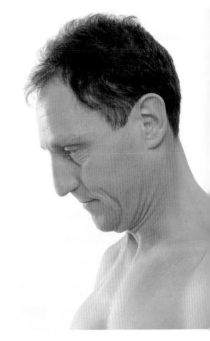

▲ Chin to chest stretch

A simple way of releasing tension stored in the muscles at the back of the neck that can be performed anywhere and at any time.

1   Slowly drop your chin down so that you are looking at the floor, without allowing your back, neck or shoulders to bend or curve.
2   Still looking at the floor, bring your chin back towards the neck so that you form a double chin. This stretches out the back of the neck.
3   Release and re-stretch several times, making sure that your shoulder and back stay upright and your chin is tucked well in to the front of the neck.

►Ear to shoulder stretch

Another simple but highly effective self-stretch for the neck, to reduce tension and stress in the muscles.

1 Sit up straight with your back upright, facing straight ahead with your chin level. This is the neutral position.
2 Slowly and gently allow the head to drop sideways so that the ear meets the shoulder. Do not twist the head – your eyes should look straight ahead the whole time and your face continue to look directly in front of you.
3 As your ear drops towards your shoulder, you should feel a stretch in the other side of the neck. Hold the stretch for at least 30 seconds before slowly raising the head back to the neutral position.
4 Repeat on the other side.

A continuation of this stretch is to move the head slightly forwards at an angle in order to allow the stretch to move further into the back of the neck:

5 Begin in the neutral position. Move your face a quarter turn to the right so that you are facing about forty-five degrees in front of you.
6 Keeping the head steady, drop the right ear towards the top of the shoulder as before, feeling a stretch around the back and side of the left side of the neck and into the top of the shoulder. Hold for 30 seconds.
7 Repeat on the left side, ear to shoulder, remembering to sit upright in the neutral position at all times to avoid twisting the neck.

tip Remember to always return to the neutral position between stretches to ensure that the neck does not twist, strain or bend.

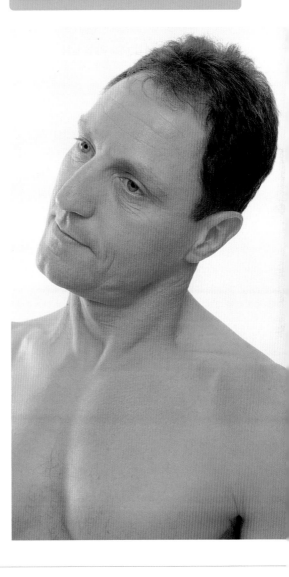

LOWER BACK PAIN can be very painful and is often due to poor posture or long hours of desk work. The following techniques can help to relieve this problem.

▼ Seated stretch with the hands between feet

To release tension in the lower back.

1   Sit up straight in a chair, facing straight ahead with your knees apart and a space of at least 1 m (3 ft) in front of you.
2   Put your arms out in front of you and slowly bend over so your head moves down between your knees and your hands travel back under the chair.
3   Stay in this stretch for several seconds before slowly returning to a sitting position.

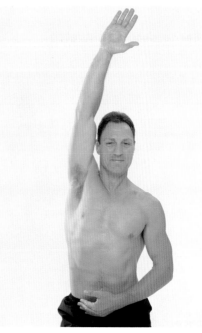

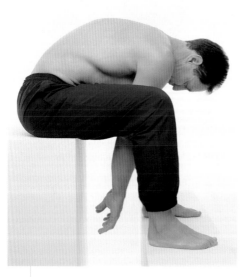

▲ Seated side stretch

To free up tension in the ribs, ease breathing and encourage relaxation, as well as stretching out the lower back by enlarging the space between vertebrae.

1   Sit up straight in a chair, facing ahead with your chin level.
2   Imagine there is a piece of string attaching your left shoulder to the ceiling. Raise your right hand straight up over your head, taking care not to squeeze the neck, and reach up as far as you can on this imaginary string.
3   Release, return to neutral and repeat a further two times breathing out as you reach upwards.
4   Repeat on the other side.

▼ Self massage of gluteals

A deep technique to ease tension in the base of the back.

1 Stand up straight and face directly ahead, with your feet hip-width apart.
2 Pull yourself up from the chest as if you were being held up by an imaginary harness (this stops pressure being put on the lower back because of sagging).
3 Place your hands on the hips with the thumbs reaching into either side of the lower back where it meets the buttocks. The fingers should rest towards the front of your body.
4 Using circular motions, massage the muscles at the top of the buttocks with your thumbs.

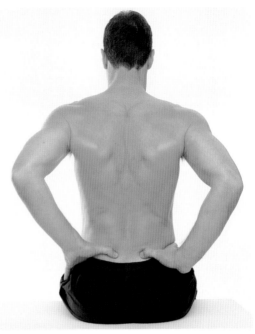

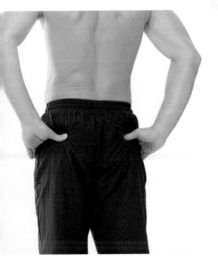

▲ Self-massage to base of spine

A simple massage technique to ease tension at the bottom of the spine and boost posture.

1 Place your hands on the lower part of the back, palms on hips, and the thumbs spread around the back facing towards each other.
2 Massage the muscles around the lower back (avoiding the spine) with the flats of your thumbs, using circular motions to cover the whole lower back.

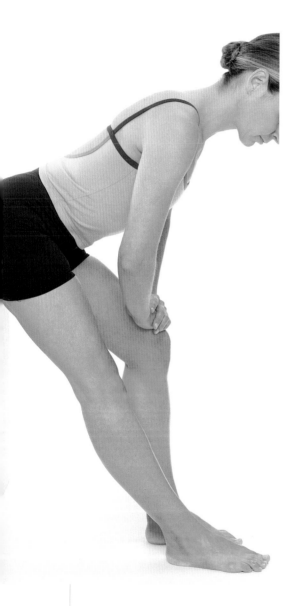

SITTING AT A DESK for hours can make the hamstring tight and stiff. These techniques will help stretch them out again.

◀ Seated hamstring stretches

To ease pressure on the lower spine by stretching out the hamstrings.

1. Sit straight on the edge of your chair facing ahead with your feet flat on the floor and your knees hip-width apart.
2. Straighten your left leg and rest the heel on the floor so that it sticks out straight in front of you.
3. Keeping your back straight and your chin in a straight line with your head (not jutting out), lean forwards over the outstretched leg until you feel a stretch in your hamstrings.
4. Hold the stretch for at least 30 seconds and repeat on the other leg.

Seated pelvic tilts

To stretch the lower back and reduce tension caused by bad posture.

1. Sit up straight with the buttocks pushed to the back of a chair and slide one hand into the curve of your lower back with the palm outwards.
2. Using the muscles in your lower abdomen and pelvis and taking extra care not to move the top of your body, which should remain totally still from the waist upwards, push your lower back against your hand and hold it there for several seconds.
3. Release the lower back and perform the stretch two or three times.

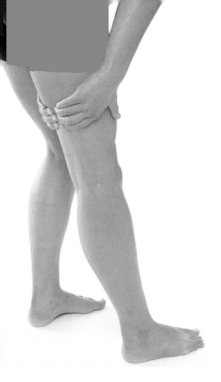

▲ Standing hamstring massage

To reduce stress in the hamstrings from over- or under-use. This simple massage technique is best performed in the shower, though it can also be used when standing normally.

1   Take your weight onto one leg with the other leg slightly bent and placed in front of you.
2   Making sure that your back stays straight, bend over from the waist so your hands reach around the back of the front thigh without stretching the shoulders, arms or back.
3   Use the fingers of both hands to knead the muscle of the back of the thigh, taking care to avoid the soft area just above the knee.
4   Repeat for the other leg.

▼ Hamstring STR

To further stretch the hamstrings and release more tension.

1   With your back straight, bend from the waist, reaching your hands around the back of your thigh.
2   Bend the knee and push two fingers of each hand (touching each other to form one point of contact) into the muscle. Push in and up towards the buttocks to stretch the hamstring.
3   Work in the stretch by slowly straightening the leg and repeat the process several times for each leg. Work around the whole thigh, but avoid the area above the knee.

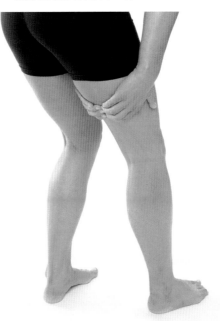

JOINT PAIN can be debilitating, but the following massages can help by boosting blood flow to the affected joint.

▼ Top of shoulder massage

To reduce tension caused by repetitive work at a desk and bad posture.

1   Place four fingers of the right hand at the midpoint between the left shoulder and neck.
2   Use a circular motion to work well into the muscle.
3   If required, work deeper by forming a hook with the fingers and drawing them to the front of the body.

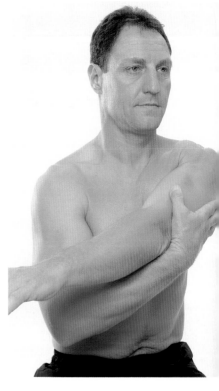

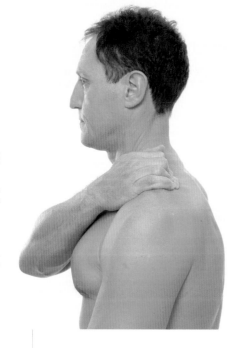

▲ Shoulder stretch across the body

To stretch out tension in the back of the shoulder and the upper arm.

1   While seated, straighten your left arm out in front of you.
2   Place the right hand across the body so the wrist touches the outside of the left arm above the elbow.
3   Looking straight ahead, use the right hand and arm to bring the left arm, still straight, across the chest to stretch out the shoulder.

▼ Deep thumb stroke of the forearm

To relieve tension in the forearm, wrist, elbow and hand.

1   While seated, place the right hand on a flat surface, such as a desk or tabletop.
2   Place the left thumb on top of the right wrist and work up towards the elbow using small strokes.
3   As a continuation of the massage, you can also work transversely, across the forearm from side to side, to work deeper into the muscle.

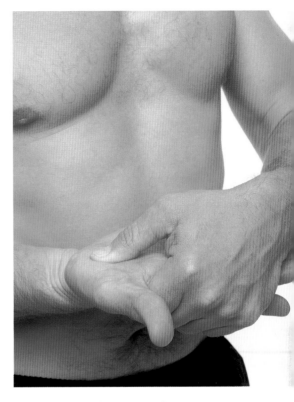

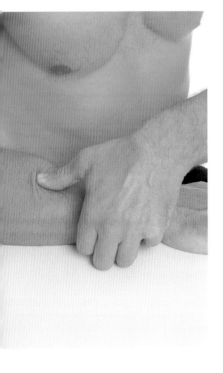

▲ Kneading the base of the thumb

To reduce tension in the hands.

1   Place the right palm upwards with the left thumb on the large pad of muscle at the base of the right thumb.
2   Using circular motions to reduce tension, work the thumb, in small strokes, from the hand to the wrist.

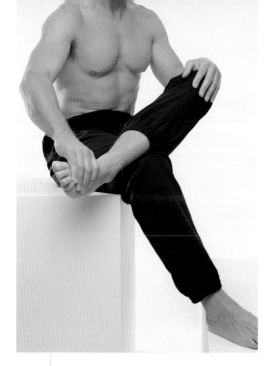

▼ Toe flexion and extension

To further boost ankle mobility and reduce tension in the lower calf.

1 Sit up straight and place the left leg across the right thigh so that the ankle rests on the knee.
2 Point the toes and stretch out the top of the foot, holding for a few seconds.
3 Using the left hand, gently bring the toes slowly up towards the shin to flex the ankle.
4 Repeat ten times, keeping movements slow and controlled.

▲ Ankle rotations

To boost flexibility and reduce stiffness in the ankle.

1 Sit up straight and place the left leg across the right thigh.
2 With the right hand gripping the left foot, rotate the ankle clockwise three times using a slow, controlled movement and not jerking or straining.
3 Rotate the ankle three times in the opposite direction.

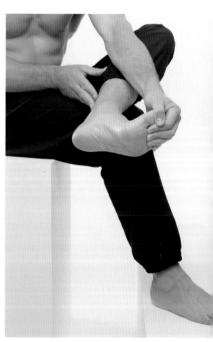

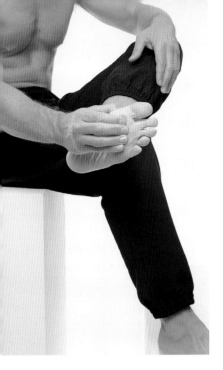

▼ Deep circular massage of the instep

To reduce tension and friction in bound-up foot tendons.

1   In the same seated position with the left foot on the right knee, work one or both thumbs on the instep (the arch) of the foot in small circular motions.
2   Continue working from the heel up the foot through to the big toe.

▲ Thumb massage to base of toes

1   Sit upright and bring the left foot onto the right knee.
2   Use the right thumb or fingers (whichever is more comfortable) to work into the base of the toes, working from the ball of the foot at the big toe towards the outside of the foot.
3   To increase the tension release, move down the foot towards the centre of the sole.

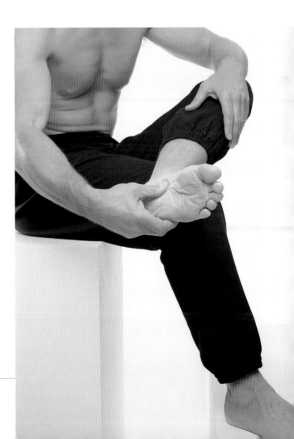

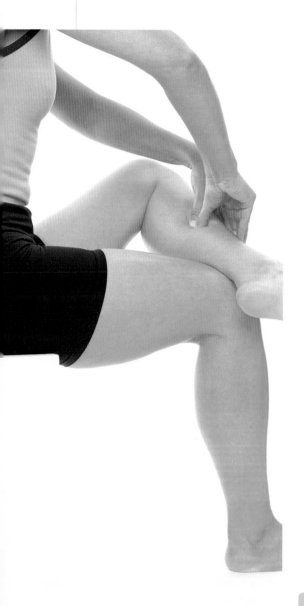

FITNESS WORKOUTS, particularly those that involve running, walking or cycling, can work the muscles of the legs very hard. You should always warm down to allow your muscles a period of gentle exercise to release toxins and reduce next-day stiffness.

These massages will help you avoid problems following a workout by targeting areas that commonly develop stiffness and soreness.

Shower self-massage

The heat and steam from the shower will boost circulation to muscles and increase the dilation of blood vessels, which can help with muscle soreness.

1   Use a hand-held showerhead to work into muscled areas like the shoulders, back, neck, thighs and calves. Make sure the temperature isn't too hot, as this can shock the skin and tissues.

◄ Compression and draw of the calf

To work out tension and blockages in the calf muscles after exercise.

1   Sit with your left foot crossed over so that it rests on the right knee.
2   Place both hands around the lower leg with thumbs facing towards you.
3   Push both thumbs down from the shin towards the floor, drawing the muscle away from the shin in a slow and controlled movement.

tip For deeper tension release, you can add active movement to this compression and draw technique. Start with the toes flexed up towards the shin and then slowly release them so they point ahead as you complete the draw.

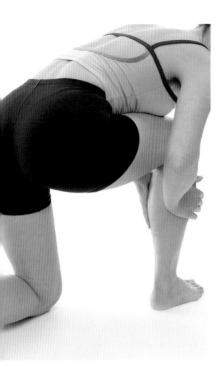

▼ Double finger draw up the shin

To reduce tension in the lower leg, particularly after walking, running, stepping or cycling.

1   Position yourself on the floor with one shin vertically in front of you.
2   Lean forwards and place the first two fingers of each hand together on the outside of the ankle joint.
3   Slowly draw your fingers up the outside of the shin towards the knee.
4   You can choose to add active muscle movement by pointing and flexing the foot as you make a second stroke.

▲ Self-compression of the calf

To get rid of toxin build-up and fluid blockage in the calf after a vigorous workout.

1   Kneel on your left knee with your right foot flat on the floor.
2   Lean forwards and place the heel of the right hand on the bottom of the right calf, as low as you feel comfortable.
3   Press into the calf muscle and hold for several seconds.
4   Move about 5 cm (2 in) up and work your way up the calf to the knee. Do not go over the same area twice.

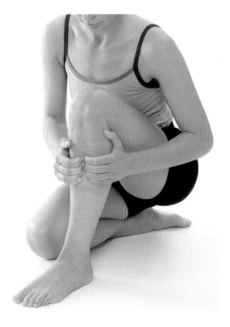

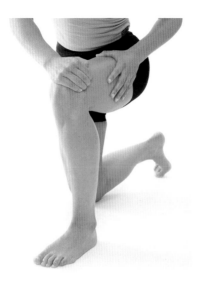

▼ Deep strokes to top of the calf

To reduce tension and pain around the top of the calf and knee.

1   In a sitting position, place both hands on either side of the calf with the thumbs at the top of the calf about 5 cm (2 in) below the knee.
2   Work both thumbs up towards the knee in deep strokes. Do not go above the crease at the back of the knee.

THESE POST-WORKOUT massages are performed in a sitting or kneeling position. You should never massage if you feel pain or discomfort anywhere in your body, or if there is any swelling or injury to the area you are treating.

▲ Transfrictional glide over the sides of the knee

To reduce tension on the knee joint following running and walking.

1   Kneel on your right knee and place the right hand over the left knee, with the fingers to the outside of the knee.
2   Working in a small, circular movement with your fingers, cover the area to the outside of the knee avoiding the kneecap.
3   For deeper contact, try adding a squeezing motion or working with the thumb.

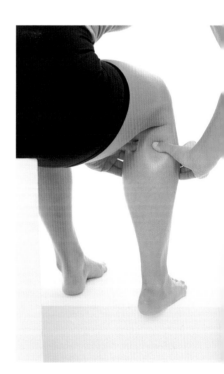

▼ STR knee

To stretch out localized areas of the thigh muscles and to release tension in the knee. Particularly good following a run or a hilly walk.

1 Sit upright and place the right thumb on the left thigh above the knee and the left thumb on top of it.
2 Straighten the leg, bringing the foot off the ground to knee level.
3 Press the thumbs into the muscle of the thigh and bring them back to your body, locking and loading the muscle.
4 Slowly lower the foot to the floor, keeping the thumb pressure constant, to deepen the stretch.
5 Move the thumbs up about 5 cm (2 in) and repeat up the whole thigh, taking care not to STR the same area twice.

▼ Calf stretch, medial and lateral

To stretch out tight calf muscles, boost toxin disposal in the lower leg and reduce stiffness.

1 Stand facing a wall, about 30 cm (1 ft) away from it.
2 Place the heel of your foot on the floor in front of the wall and the ball of your foot against the wall so that the toes point up towards the shin.
3 Keeping the leg straight, bring the thigh and the knee towards the wall to stretch the calf. Hold the stretch for at least 30 seconds.
4 To spread the stretch further into the calf, move the heel a little to the right of centre and repeat the stretch, then repeat about 5 cm (2in) to the left. Note that your toes stay in the same place for all three stretches, it's only your heel that moves sideways.

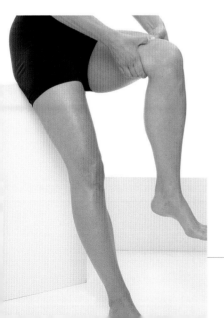

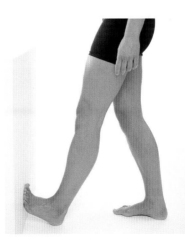

THE FOLLOWING TECHNIQUES target areas that are particularly affected by tension.

▼ Anterior chest massage

To reduce tension across the front chest, to free up breathing and loosen the neck.

1   Place the four fingers of your right hand on the left side of your chest.
2   Starting at the centre of the chest, move the fingers in a circular motion working out towards the shoulder.
3   Breathe in and out slowly as you perform the massage, deepening the strokes lightly as you breathe out.

▼ Anterior neck stretch

To work further into the chest and front of the neck.

1   Use four fingers in circular motions as before, but this time turn your head to the right so that you stretch out the muscles and ligaments at the front of the neck.

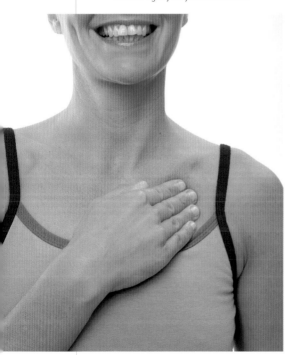
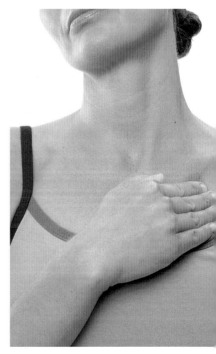

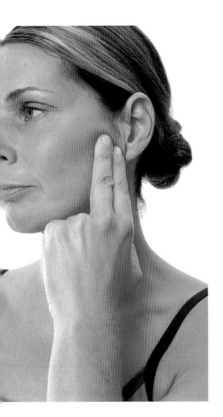

▼ Scalp tension buster

To reduce tension held in the scalp and to boost relaxation.

1　Spread out the fingers and thumbs of both hands and place them at either side of the head, with the thumbs above the ears and towards the back of the neck.
2　Work the fingers and thumbs in small circular motions.
3　After a few seconds, move the hands so that they cover a different area.
4　Breathe deeply in and out to enhance the relaxation.

▲ Two finger massage to base of jaw

To relieve tension in the jaw and sides of the face.

1　Place the two fingers of the left hand together on the jaw so that the first finger fits into the bony area in front of the earlobe.
2　Using small circular motions, work the thumb lightly into the jaw area, keeping the contact broad and being careful not to press too hard. The jaw should move slightly to the side.

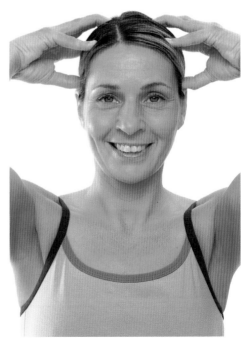

THE FOLLOWING HAND-MASSAGE techniques are designed for you to do at work to protect against stress, tension build-up and Repetitive Strain Injury (RSI).

Sit correctly for muscle balance. As a general rule, good posture can help prevent injury and reduce tension in all the muscles of your body, as well as aid concentration and mental acuity. If sitting for some time, periodically check that you are in the right position (see notes, opposite). If you have trouble remembering, try fixing a memory aid, like a red spot sticker, somewhere on your desk and checking your posture every time you catch sight of it.

▼ Compressions to back of hand

To reduce tension in the hand from dextrous, repetitive work such as writing and typing.

1　Place the left hand in front of you, palm down.
2　Using the right thumb, press into the back of your left hand, holding the stretch for a few seconds each.
3　Move the compressions around taking care not to cover the same area twice.

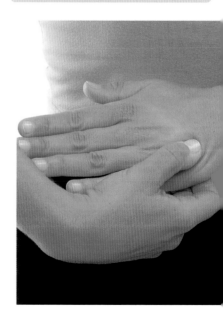

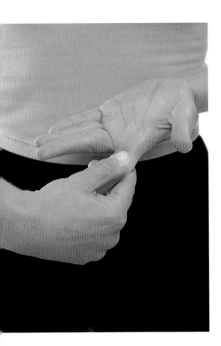

▼ Wrist, forearm and hand stretch

To release tension in the whole of the lower arm and hand.

1   Hold your left hand out in front of you, keeping your arm straight.
2   Use your right hand to bring the palm and fingers back so that you feel a stretch in your forearm. Hold for at least 30 seconds.

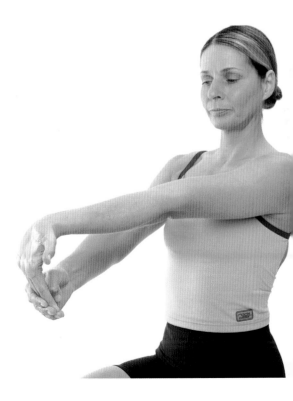

▲ Thumb compressions through the fingers

To reduce tension in the thumb and wrist.

1   Place the left hand in front of you, palm up.
2   Press the thumb into the bottom of the first finger, working your way up the finger so that you press into each of the three sections.
3   Work your way down each finger, repeating the three compressions.

THE FOLLOWING TECHNIQUES help to aid
common abdominal problems.

▼ Period pain

**Helps to combat menstrual pain, as well
as soreness due to muscle cramp.**

1   Sit or stand with your lower back free.
2   Place your hands on your hips with
    the thumbs on the lower back at hip
    level on either side of the spine.
3   Move the thumbs in small, light
    circular motions into the pressure
    points of the lower back. Stop if you
    feel any discomfort.

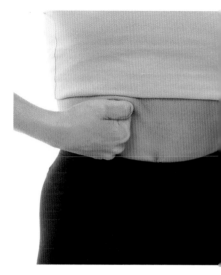

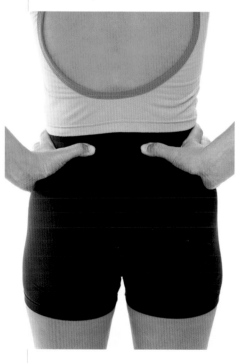

▲ Wind pains

**To reduce pain caused by the build up
of wind in the abdomen by releasing
trapped air and boosting digestive flow.**

1   Find a quiet spot where you won't be
    embarrassed if wind escapes.
2   Stand or sit comfortably.
3   Form a loose fist with your right
    fingers (so that the palm stays flat but
    the fingers are curled) and place it at
    the front of the right hip.
4   Use loose circular motions in a
    clockwise motion to follow the line
    of the large intestine, working up
    the right side to the ribs, across
    the bottom of the ribcage and
    down towards the left hip.

Using acupressure

One or two fingers should be used to stimulate each acupressure relief point using constant pressure. Circular massage movements should not be used. Initially, keep the pressure light and constant for 30 seconds, then repeat the compression with more pressure if required. Each compression should be held for 30 seconds.

Acupressure point 1

An instant mood-booster point to help fight depression and lift the spirit. This is found where the thumb and forefinger form a V. Use the opposite thumb to push into the area.

Acupressure point 2

A tension-relief point, good for relieving tension headaches, boosting concentration and relieving tired eyes. Found in the occipital hollow where the bottom of the skull meets the neck, either side of the spine. Use the thumb to gently press either side of this area.

Acupressure point 3

A stress-relieving point that is good for reducing anxiety and tension. Found at the top-centre of the forearm in the large muscle just below the crease of the elbow.

Acupressure point 4

A metabolism-boosting point, good for chest and eye problems and boosting general circulation and metabolism. Found on top of the foot, roughly in line with the middle two toes and directly over the arch.

Acupressure point 5

An immune-boosting point, good for combating fatigue and depression. Found on the inside of the ankle above the foot between the Achilles tendon and the anklebone.

Acupressure point 6

A point for pain relief, tension release and mood-boosting. Found on the back, in line with the kidneys. Sit up straight in a chair and form a fist with each hand. Place the fists behind your back, level with the elbow, and lean back gently to stimulate the point.

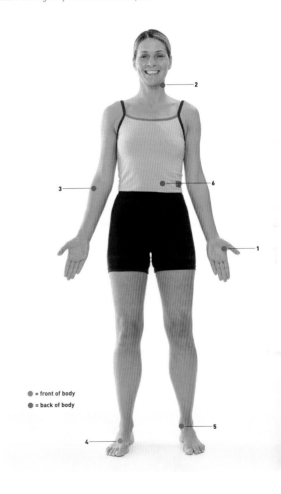

● = front of body
● = back of body

Body Therapy
and Aftercare

The period of time after massage is very important for ensuring maximum therapeutic benefits for the body and mind. This chapter shows you how to take the best care of your physical and mental states between massages in order to maximize the benefits and ensure that your feeling of wellbeing lasts.

Massage not only relaxes and unwinds tension, it also acts as a detoxifier, soothes away problems in the body's soft tissues and boosts circulation and lymphatic drainage. But the benefits do not have to stop when the massage is over. Making a few small changes could have far-reaching benefits for your whole health.

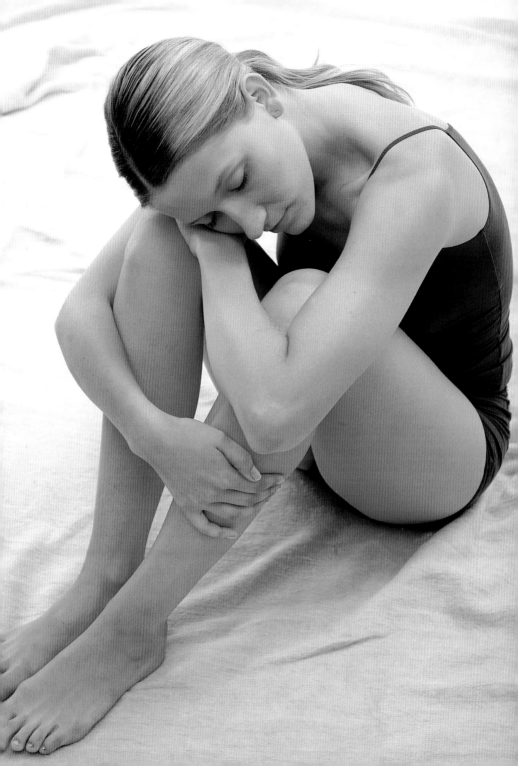

Making the most of massage

Massage can sometimes elicit an emotional response. When toxins and tension trapped in the body are released, fears, anxiety and sadness may come to the surface. Some people feel sleepy, faint or light-headed immediately afterwards and may need a little time to readjust to the pace of normal life. Take care if you're driving right after a massage, as deep relaxation may cause reaction time to slow down. Never drive if you feel light-headed or sleepy; sit quietly or have a snooze and wait until you feel ready to drive.

On rare occasions there may be a physical response like headache, feeling hot, mild nausea or perspiration. However, these symptoms are usually only experienced during the first few massages or in people who haven't had a massage for a long time. They should disappear quickly with rest.

Detoxify

Avoid drinking alcohol or caffeine or smoking for at least 12 hours after to help your body continue the detoxification process. Adding toxins like alcohol or nicotine could adversely affect the process. Regular massage will help your body cope with everyday toxins, and keeping it as free of toxins as possible before and after a massage will help you stay healthy long-term.

Sleep like a baby

One of the major side-effects of massage is a feeling of tiredness – as toxins are released the body can become profoundly heavy. If your body feels fatigued during or after massage, don't fight it. Giving in to tiredness is a luxury we do not often allow ourselves. If you feel sleepy afterwards, it is because your body is telling you it needs to slow down.

Visualization

While the massage is in progress, close your eyes and think of a place that makes you feel comforted, relaxed and calm – it could be a perfect landscape, a gentle lake at sunset or a favourite view – then mentally transport yourself there with all your senses. Think about how the place smells, feels and sounds as well as what you see. While you visualize this special, timeless place, allow your breathing to become deeper and rhythmic and let worries and tension flood away. Take time to bring yourself slowly back to the present, concentrating on what is going on around you, before you open your eyes.

Keep it light

Avoid eating or drinking heavily straight after a massage, or engaging in physical activity. This could divert energy away from vital healing processes toward digestion – steer clear of stimulants like caffeine and stick to water or herbal tea, light snacks and fresh fruit. Make sure you drink enough water to avoid the dehydration that can follow massage. Water keeps the body working efficiently, gives the lymph and circulation systems a helping hand and plumps up skin, making it look and feel fresh and young.

Boost circulation

Slow circulation can affect your body's systems and make the skin dull, dry and flaky. Massage helps circulation but there is also a lot that you can do for yourself in between massages. Use a body buffer or loofah in the shower to rub dry skin off your legs and arms, remembering to work from the extremities towards the heart. Slight redness of the skin is a sign that the blood is flowing strongly to the surface.

Warm down

A post-exercise warming down will help prevent cramp, injury and muscle soreness, as it helps your muscles rid themselves of toxins. Aim for at least five to ten minutes of gentle exercise to end your workout.

Think tall

Good posture can help you get through life without pain and injury. Try to think about how you sit or stand. If you are still for long periods of time – sitting at a desk, cooking or watching television – aim to keep your spine in the neutral position, which will help to reduce stress on the back.

Take a break

Giving a massage can be very draining on your energy levels so, after you have given someone a massage, make sure you take some time to recharge your own batteries. Make sure you drink plenty of water and avoid rushing on to the next thing. Allow your body ten minutes of relaxation and renewal, sitting or lying somewhere quiet and calm.

Vitamin boost

You should aim to eat at least five portions of fruit and vegetables every day to boost your intake of vitamins, minerals and anti-oxidants. Vitamins A, B and C, found in abundance in tomatoes, fruit, leafy green vegetables and watercress, are particularly important for a healthy diet.

Essential nutrients

Fatty acids and elements like zinc and calcium are essential for strong skin, bones, hair and nails. Seafood, leafy green vegetables and nuts all contain these nutritious elements and will help to keep your skin in top condition. Consuming oily fish like mackerel and salmon ensures you have the right building blocks for all-round health.

Antioxidize yourself

Pollution, toxins, alcohol, smoking and stress can lead to a build-up of free radicals in the body, which, if left unchecked, can cause long-term damage. To combat this, make sure you include free-radical busting anti-oxidants in your diet; these are found in fresh fruit and vegetables, garlic, onions and nuts and seeds.

Glossary

The following conditions may be helped using the massage techniques detailed in this book.

Arthritis

Sore joints can be soothed by boosting circulation through massage:
- Compressions to back of hand (page 116)
- Thumb compressions through the fingers (page 117)
- Thumb massage to base of toes (page 109)
- Deep circular massage of the instep (page 109)
(Never massage if arthritis is acute or inflamed – this could be painful and even make it worse.)

Asthma and breathing problems

Tension in the muscles around the ribs, abdomen and chest can worsen the symptoms of asthma. Try the following to relax the trunk and breathing muscles:
- Anterior chest massage (page 114)
- Diaphragm STR (page 92)
- Deep finger rib effleurage (page 92)
- Acupressure point 4 (page 119)

Blocked sinuses

Swollen or blocked sinuses can cause problems with headaches, stuffiness and tiredness. Try the following to clear away excess fluids and help drain your sinuses so you can breathe easy:
- Circular sinus compressions (page 98)
- Occiput pressure release (page 41)

Cellulite

There is some evidence that massage can help clear away cellulite. Try effleurage techniques on the thighs and calves to boost lymphatic drainage and increase blood flow to the skin:
- Thigh effleurage I and II (page 73)
- Self massage of gluteals (page 103)
- Thigh petrissage (page 74)

Circulation

Boost circulation and lymphatic drainage using the following general techniques:
- Effleurage and petrissage of the arms (pages 62–70)
- Effleurage and petrissage of the legs (pages 73–83)
- Acupressure point 4 (page 119)

Concentration

Tired muscles and aches and pains can not only make the body weary but also distract the mind. Boost your concentration with these massages:
- Temple massage (page 98)
- Anterior neck stretch (page 114)
- Acupressure points 2 and 4 (page 119)

Depression

Help your body to combat depression by using finger massage:
- Acupressure points 1 and 5 (page 119)

Eyestrain

Soothe tired eyes using these facial massages:
- Occiput draw (page 99)
- Chin to chest stretch (page 100)
- Ear to shoulder stretch (page 101)

Fatigue

Help the body to combat fatigue by giving yourself a rejuvenating metabolism boost using the following simple techniques:
- Complete arm shake for relaxation (page 70)
- Complete leg relaxation vibrations (page 83)
- Acupressure points 2 and 5 (page 119)
- Occiput pressure release (page 41)

Hangover

Headaches, upset stomachs and tired muscles the morning after can be soothed using:
- Temple massage (page 98)
- Scalp tension buster (page 115)
- Occiput pressure release (page 41)
- Alternate hands effleurage (page 90)

Headaches

Reduce pain using the following techniques:
- Occiput draw (page 99)
- Occiput pressure release (page 41)
- Scalp tension buster (page 115)

Indigestion

Dyspepsia can be uncomfortable and painful. Try the following chest and abdominal techniques:
- Clavicular effleurage (page 38)
- Sternal effleurage (page 39)
- Alternate hands effleurage (page 90)

Insomnia

Sometimes insomnia is made worse by tension and muscle stiffness in the body, so try these relaxing, sleep-inducing techniques to help you drop off:
- Massages to neck and shoulder (pages 40, 43, 44–47)
- Complete back relaxation stroke (pages 54–55)
- Acupressure point 3 (page 119)

Stiff knees

This complaint is often caused by tightness and rigidity in the muscles surrounding the knee. Free up the knee joint using the following techniques:
- Thigh effleurage I and II (page 73)
- Hamstrings effleurage I (page 79)
- Self-compression of the calf (page 111)
- Calf stretch, medial and lateral (page 113)

Lower back pain

The lower back is a common place for pain, especially among people with bad posture and weak core strength. The following may reduce pain and stiffness:
- Acupressure point 6 (page 119)
- Self-massage to base of spine (page 103)
- Transverse draw of gluteals (page 52)

Neck stiffness

Stiffness in the neck area, especially if caused by bad posture, can be reduced using the following techniques to reduce toxin build-up in muscles and boost flexibility:
- Chin to chest stretch (page 100)
- Ear to shoulder stretch (page 101)
- Top of shoulder massage (page 106)

Period Pain

Monthly cramps can be helped by warming up the area above the front of the hips (see page 118) and by performing:
- Deep thumb lower back effleurage (page 49)
- Acupressure point 6 (page 119)

Relaxation

All massage can be relaxing if a light but firm touch is used, but these are particularly beneficial for a quick fix:
- Complete back relaxation stroke (pages 54–55)
- Scalp tension buster (page 115)
- Vibrations to arms and legs (pages 70 and 83)

RSI (Repetitive Strain Injury)

Repetitive Strain Injury, now fairly common among office workers who use keyboards all day, is a condition that affects mainly the forearms. Reduce pain and discomfort using the following techniques:
- STR of forearm and tricep (pages 67 and 68)
- Wrist, forearm and hand stretch (page 117)
- Kneading the base of the thumb (page 107)

Stomach ache

Pains and aches caused by muscle spasms in the digestive tract can sometimes be soothed by gentle massage to the area:
- Alternate hands effleurage (page 90)
- Kneading of the abdomen (page 93)

(You should not massage if the pain is severe or if massage makes it worse)

Stress relief

Any massage aids stress relief, but the following massages are particularly useful, especially if essential oils are used:
- Complete back relaxation stroke (pages 54–55)
- Scalp tension buster (page 115)
- Acupressure points 3 and 5 (page 119)

(See limitations for essential oil use on pages 18–19)

Swollen ankles / feet

Massages that boost circulation in the legs can help the lymphatic system to drain away excess fluid. Combine the following massages with elevating the affected areas for reduction of swelling:
- Calf effleurage I and II (page 82)
- Hamstring effleurage I (page 79)
- Toe flexion and extension (page 108)

Tooth grinding

Grinding the teeth, especially at night, can cause jaw, neck and head pain as a result of muscle soreness and spasm. Soothe it away with the following massages:
- Two finger massage to base of jaw (page 115)
- Occiput draw (page 99)

Wind Pains

Get rid of wind using basic abdominal massage techniques (or see page 118):
- Clockwise circular stroking (pages 88–89)

Index

Resources

Reading

Atkinson, Mary, Hand and Foot Massage, London, Carlton, 2001.
Specializes on the caring aspect of massage.

Atkinson, Mary, Indian Head Massage, London, Carlton, 2000.
Expert Mary Atkinson teaches the traditional Ayurvedic head-massage method.

Cash, Mel, Sport and Remedial Massage Therapy, London, Ebury, 1996.
This is an excellent book for massage therapy students.

Cash, Mel, and Ylinen, Jan, Sport's Massage, London, Hutchinson, 1998
This is a great reference for all aspects of sports massage techniques.

Norris, Chris, Back Stability, Human Kinetics, 2002.
Physiotherapist Chris Norris looks at posture and the muscles around the spine.

Sanderson, Mary, Soft Tissue Release: A Practical Handbook for Physical Therapists, Corpus Publishing, 2002.
An in-depth look at STR techniques.

Organizations

American Institute of Massage Therapy
1570 Brookhollow Drive, Suite 200, Santa Ana, California 92705, USA; tele: 714 432 7879; www.aimtinc.com; info@ aimtinc.com. A California-based massage school for accredited sports massage training.

American Massage Therapy Association
820 Davis Street, Suite 100, Evanston, Illinois, 60201–4464, USA; tele: 847 864 0123; www.amtamassage.org. Represents 46,000 massage therapists in 27 countries, and funds and reports on the latest research.

International Massage Association
www.imagroup.com
A database of massage therapists from all over the world with links to the healing arts. Please note that the IMA is not a regulatory body.

London School of Sports Massage
28 Station Parade, Willesden Green, London NW2 4NX, England; tele: 0208 452 8855; www.lssm.com. Runs weekend courses at Regent's College, London.

Southern School of Massage Therapy
Paul Wills is the founder of the Southern Massage School, based in Kingston, Surrey, England, which trains massage therapists. For more information tele: 07816 834 705 or search www.ssmt.net.

Sports Massage Association
PO Box 44347, London SW19 1WD, England; tele: 020 8545 0861; info@ thesma.org; www.sportsmassageassociation.org. A new body designed to promote and regulate sports massage in the UK. Contact to locate a practitioner.

Acknowledgements

Paul Wills would like to thank Don and Mary Crane, Sam Powell and Suzanne Burnett.